CANCER ETIOLOGY, DIAGNOSIS AND TREATMENTS

NEW RESEARCH ON HEMATOLOGICAL MALIGNANCIES

CANCER ETIOLOGY, DIAGNOSIS AND TREATMENTS

Additional books and e-books in this series can be found on Nova's website under the Series tab.

CANCER ETIOLOGY, DIAGNOSIS AND TREATMENTS

NEW RESEARCH ON HEMATOLOGICAL MALIGNANCIES

DAVID K. GIOIA
EDITOR

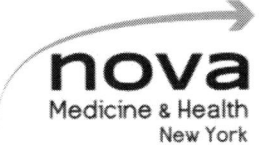

Copyright © 2021 by Nova Science Publishers, Inc.

All rights reserved. No part of this book may be reproduced, stored in a retrieval system or transmitted in any form or by any means: electronic, electrostatic, magnetic, tape, mechanical photocopying, recording or otherwise without the written permission of the Publisher.

We have partnered with Copyright Clearance Center to make it easy for you to obtain permissions to reuse content from this publication. Simply navigate to this publication's page on Nova's website and locate the "Get Permission" button below the title description. This button is linked directly to the title's permission page on copyright.com. Alternatively, you can visit copyright.com and search by title, ISBN, or ISSN.

For further questions about using the service on copyright.com, please contact:
Copyright Clearance Center
Phone: +1-(978) 750-8400   Fax: +1-(978) 750-4470   E-mail: info@copyright.com

NOTICE TO THE READER

The Publisher has taken reasonable care in the preparation of this book, but makes no expressed or implied warranty of any kind and assumes no responsibility for any errors or omissions. No liability is assumed for incidental or consequential damages in connection with or arising out of information contained in this book. The Publisher shall not be liable for any special, consequential, or exemplary damages resulting, in whole or in part, from the readers' use of, or reliance upon, this material. Any parts of this book based on government reports are so indicated and copyright is claimed for those parts to the extent applicable to compilations of such works.

Independent verification should be sought for any data, advice or recommendations contained in this book. In addition, no responsibility is assumed by the Publisher for any injury and/or damage to persons or property arising from any methods, products, instructions, ideas or otherwise contained in this publication.

This publication is designed to provide accurate and authoritative information with regard to the subject matter covered herein. It is sold with the clear understanding that the Publisher is not engaged in rendering legal or any other professional services. If legal or any other expert assistance is required, the services of a competent person should be sought. FROM A DECLARATION OF PARTICIPANTS JOINTLY ADOPTED BY A COMMITTEE OF THE AMERICAN BAR ASSOCIATION AND A COMMITTEE OF PUBLISHERS.

Additional color graphics may be available in the e-book version of this book.

Library of Congress Cataloging-in-Publication Data

ISBN: 978-1-53619-955-0

Published by Nova Science Publishers, Inc. † New York

CONTENTS

Preface vii

Chapter 1 Molecular and Cytogenetic Markers
and their Clinical Implications
in Myeloproliferative Neoplasms 1
Seda Ekizoglu and Onur Baykara

Chapter 2 Treatment of Myeloid Hematologic Malignancies
with Isocitrate Dehydrogenase Mutations
by Inhibitors of this Enzyme 51
Ota Fuchs

Chapter 3 Inhibition of Nuclear Export as a New Therapy
in Hematologic Malignancies 89
Ota Fuchs

Chapter 4 Poly(ADP-Ribose) Polymerase Inhibitors
in the Treatment of Myelodysplastic
Syndrome and Acute Myeloid Leukemia 113
Ota Fuchs

Index 139

Preface

Hematological malignancies, defined as cancers that affect the blood, bone marrow, and lymph nodes, represent a serious health care challenge for oncologists. Chapter One focuses on cytogenetic and molecular markers and summarizes their importance in identification, treatment and prognosis in patients with myeloproliferative neoplasms. Chapter Two details the efficacy of treatment of myeloid hematologic malignancies with isocitrate dehydrogenase mutations by inhibitors of this enzyme. Chapter Three describes the use of Selinexor and other drugs for the treatment of hematologic malignancies. Chapter Four explains the utility of poly(ADP-ribose) polymerase inhibitors in the treatment of myelodysplastic syndrome and acute myeloid leukemia.

Chapter 1 - Myeloproliferative neoplasms (MPNs) are clonal disorders of the hematopoietic stem cells that are characterized by increased proliferation of erythroid, megakaryocytic, or granulocytic cells in the bone marrow that is associated with increased peripheral blood parameters. According to the revised World Health Organization (WHO) classification (2016), MPNs include chronic myeloid leukemia (CML), chronic neutrophilic leukemia (CNL), polycythemia vera (PV), primary myelofibrosis (PMF), essential thrombocythemia (ET), chronic eosinophilic leukemia [not otherwise specified (NOS)] and MPN-unclassifiable (MPN-U). This classification is based on the morphology of the cell, as well as the clinical and genetic features of each disease. Many molecular and cytogenetic abnormalities have been identified for the pathogenesis of these diseases. Chromosomal aberrations such as total or partial trisomy, deletion, unbalanced translocation and rarely balanced translocation and somatic mutations detected in MPNs affect the expression of some tumor suppressor genes and/or oncogenes resulting in initiation and/or progression of the disease. It is of major importance to detect these abnormalities for differential diagnosis, follow-up of the patient and prognosis of the disease. Therefore, the physician should consider evaluating the laboratory and clinical findings together to achieve the best outcome. The aim of this chapter is to focus on cytogenetic and molecular markers and summarize their importance in identification, treatment and prognosis in patients with MPNs.

Chapter 2 - Isocitrate dehydrogenase (IDH) is an important metabolic enzyme in the Krebs Cycle that catalyzes the conversion of isocitrate to α-ketoglutarate. The mutant IDH protein leads to an accumulation of 2-hydroxyglutarate, a metabolite with oncogenic activity via epigenetic mechanisms. This metabolite is similar to α-ketoglutarate and competitively inhibits α-ketoglutarate-dependent enzymes, alters DNA and histone methylation, and impairs cellular growth and differentiation. Recurrent IDH1 and IDH2 mutations occur in about 20% of patients with acute myeloid leukemia (AML) and 5% of patients with myelodysplastic syndromes (MDS). Small molecule inhibitors of mutant IDH1 and IDH2 were developed and used in pre-clinical and clinical studies. Two of these inhibitors, ivosidenib (AG-120, Tibsovo) and enasidenib (AG-221, Idhifa) were approved by the US Food and Drug Administration (FDA) for the treatment of newly diagnosed and relapsed/refractory IDH1 and IDH2 mutant AML, respectively. Despite the high efficacy and activity of these IDH1 and IDH2 inhibitors, monotherapy showed response rates of less than 50%. Resistance was described in some cases with co-occurring mutations in receptor tyrosine kinase FLT3, transcription factors (RUNX1, GATA-2, CEBPA), or IDH1 second-site mutation. Therefore, various therapies that use a combination of the IDH1 and IDH2 inhibitors with hypomethylating agent azacitidine were studied with better results than when monotherapy was used.

Chapter 3 - A nuclear-cytoplasmic transport plays an important role in the development of cancer and drug resistance. Exportin 1 (XPO1) is the major mammalian nuclear export receptor protein, also known as chromosome maintenance 1 (CRM1). XPO1 interacts with Ras-related nuclear protein and with nucleoporins in the nuclear pore complex and transports multiple tumor suppressor proteins (eg p53, FOXO, p21 pRB, BRCA1/2), growth regulators, and oncoprotein mRNAs (eg c-myc, Bcl-xL, MDM2, cyclins) containing a leucine-rich nuclear export signal (NES). XPO1 is also involved in the regulation of cytoplasmic localization and translation of c-myc and other oncoprotein mRNAs (eg cyclin D1, Bcl-6, Mdm2, and Pim) through complexing with eukaryotic initiation factor 4E (eIF4E). The XPO1 protein level is increased in many types of cancer including hematological malignancies (multiple myeloma. diffuse large B-cell lymphoma, chronic lymphocytic leukemia, mantle cell lymphoma, T-cell lymphoma, myelodysplastic syndrome, and acute myeloid leukemia). As a result of the increased nuclear-cytoplasmic transport in cancer cells, an elevated level of multiple tumor suppressor proteins and oncoproteins in the cytoplasm leads to advanced disease, resistance to therapy, and poor survival. Thus, XPO1 is a promising cancer drug target. Selinexor (XPOVIO) is the first member of small molecule oral inhibitors of exportin 1 developed for the treatment of cancer. Eltanexor, also known as KPT-8602 or ATG-016, is a member of the second generation of these inhibitors and its anti-leukemic activity was successfully demonstrated in pre-clinical models of acute myeloid leukemia and acute lymphoblastic leukemia. Eltanexor is presently studied in clinical trials in patients with relapsed or refractory multiple myeloma (RRMM) and with intermediate and higher risk myelodysplastic syndrome. Selinexor in combination with synthetic glucocorticoid dexamethasone was approved by the United States Food and Drug Administration (USFDA) on July 3, 2019, for the treatment of adult patients with RRMM who have received at least four prior therapies. Selinexor in combination with bortezomib and dexamethasone was approved in December 2020 for the treatment of adult patients with multiple myeloma who have received at least one prior therapy. Selinexor was also approved by USFDA for the treatment of adult patients with relapsed or refractory diffuse large B-cell lymphoma after at least two lines of systemic therapy. Selinexor is also studied in clinical trials in other hematologic malignancies.

Chapter 4 - The Poly(ADP-ribose) polymerase (PARP) family of 18 proteins has important functions in cellular processes such as the regulation of chromatin remodeling, transcription, apoptosis, stress response, and DNA damage response. PARP-1 is a critical DNA repair enzyme in the base excision repair pathway and an attractive target in cancer therapy. Lynparza (olaparib) and other PARP inhibitors (PARPi) had anti-proliferative and pro-apoptotic effects in human acute myeloid leukemia (AML) blasts at concentrations that do not affect the viability of normal bone marrow stem cells. Although PARPi can generally slow leukemic cell growth, PARPi treatment of RUNX1-RUNXT1, promyelocytic leukemia-retinoic acid receptor-α (PML-RARα) fusion genes bearing AML cells resulted in their morphological differentiation into monocytic and granulocytic lineages, which was consistent with leukemic differentiation induced by excessive DNA damage. These chromosomal translocations could weaken the homologous recombination repair activity and sensitize AML cells to PARPi treatment. Olaparib cytotoxicity on primary AML blasts was caused by drug-induced DNA damage, upregulation of death receptors, and transcription factor NF-κB activation. PARP inhibitors induced anti-leukemic effects also in *FLT3-ITD* AML, where PARPi and FLT3 inhibitors showed synergistic effect. *IDH* mutations also sensitize AML cells to PARP inhibitors. PARP contributes to immune evasion of anti-tumor immune cells by PARP-dependent apoptosis through increased reactive oxygen species (ROS) and by PARP-mediated downregulation of natural killer cell-activating receptor-ligand (NKG2DL) expression on AML cells. PARPi reversed the ROS-induced apoptosis of NK and T cells. High-risk myelodysplastic syndrome (MDS) cases are associated with a decrease of apoptosis and high levels of genomic instability caused by alterations in DNA damage response pathways. Olaparib as a single agent or in combination with hypomethylating agents (decitabine or azacitidine) was not only cytotoxic, but also stimulated differentiation of immature MDS myeloid cells. Recently, proteolysis targeting chimera (PROTAC) for PARP-1 degradation was designed.

In: New Research on Hematological ... ISBN: 978-1-53619-955-0
Editor: David K. Gioia © 2021 Nova Science Publishers, Inc.

Chapter 1

MOLECULAR AND CYTOGENETIC MARKERS AND THEIR CLINICAL IMPLICATIONS IN MYELOPROLIFERATIVE NEOPLASMS

Seda Ekizoglu[*]*, PhD and Onur Baykara, PhD*
Istanbul University-Cerrahpasa, Cerrahpasa Medical Faculty,
Department of Medical Biology, Istanbul, Turkey

ABSTRACT

Myeloproliferative neoplasms (MPNs) are clonal disorders of the hematopoietic stem cells that are characterized by increased proliferation of erythroid, megakaryocytic, or granulocytic cells in the bone marrow that is associated with increased peripheral blood parameters. According to the revised World Health Organization (WHO) classification (2016), MPNs include chronic myeloid leukemia (CML), chronic neutrophilic leukemia (CNL), polycythemia vera (PV), primary myelofibrosis (PMF), essential thrombocythemia (ET), chronic eosinophilic leukemia [not otherwise specified (NOS)] and MPN-unclassifiable (MPN-U). This classification is based on the morphology of the cell, as well as the clinical and genetic features of each disease.

---

[*] Corresponding Author's E-mail: ekizoglu.seda@gmail.com

Many molecular and cytogenetic abnormalities have been identified for the pathogenesis of these diseases. Chromosomal aberrations such as total or partial trisomy, deletion, unbalanced translocation and rarely balanced translocation and somatic mutations detected in MPNs affect the expression of some tumor suppressor genes and/or oncogenes resulting in initiation and/or progression of the disease. It is of major importance to detect these abnormalities for differential diagnosis, follow-up of the patient and prognosis of the disease. Therefore, the physician should consider evaluating the laboratory and clinical findings together to achieve the best outcome. The aim of this chapter is to focus on cytogenetic and molecular markers and summarize their importance in identification, treatment and prognosis in patients with MPNs.

INTRODUCTION

An average person has about 5 liters of blood. Blood has essential roles in living organisms such as delivering nutrients (vitamins, minerals, fats and sugars) and oxygen to the cells and tissues. The waste products are transferred to the liver and kidneys, and carbon dioxide is carried to the lungs with a very efficient circulatory system. In addition, it helps the body fight against the pathogens through the immune system and regulates the metabolism via endocrine system.

Blood consists of main components which are red blood cells (RBCs, erythrocytes), white blood cells (WBCs, leukocytes), platelets (thrombocytes), and plasma. In human body, there are about 4-5 million RBCs per microliter in women and 5-6 million in men. They are produced in the red bone marrow with a special process called erythropoiesis that lasts about seven days. The diameter of an erythrocyte is approximately 6-8 µm and the shape is a biconcave disk. At any given time, human body has about 20-30 trillion RBCs and the life span of each RBC is about 120 days. RBCs contain hemoglobin, an abundantly found protein in the RBCs that carries oxygen and iron to the cells and tissues. They also take the carbon dioxide from the tissues to the lungs.

White blood cells are the main components of the immune system, which fight against the infectious agents, such as bacteria and viruses.

Unlike the RBCs and platelets, they have a nucleus. The WBCs are produced in the bone marrow and their origin is hematopoietic stem cells, which are then differentiated to produce the five major types of WBCs: neutrophils, eosinophils and basophils (granulocytes), and lymphocytes and monocytes (agranulocytes). In addition, the WBCs can be classified into other subgroups, such as lymphocytes (B lymphocytes, named after being produced in bone marrow cells or bursa), T cells (named after being produced in thymus cells) and natural killer (NK) cells. An average healthy person has approximately 4,000-10,000 WBCs per microliter of blood and a WBC count that is lower or higher than this range may be an indicator of a disease.

Platelets are one of the main components of blood that function in blood clot formation, thus prevention of bleeding. Like WBCs, they are anucleated, biconvex discoid shaped cells, with a diameter of 2-3 μm. An average person has about 150,000-500,000 per cubic millimeter. They take their origin from the myeloid stem cells and megakaryocytes and thrombopoietin (TPO) regulates the production. The platelets have an average life span of 8-9 days, and since they function in blood clot formation, any inconsistency in this tightly regulated system may cause some blood disorders.

Blood plasma is the liquid component of the blood that is responsible for carrying proteins and the cells via the circulatory system. About half of the total body volume is blood plasma and is mainly made of water (approx. 95%), and contains many different molecules such as blood clotting factors, hormones, electrolytes, proteins, oxygen and carbon dioxide. A balanced blood plasma is essential for electrolyte concentration and immune system activity. All these factors and mechanisms are strictly controlled by the cell and DNA and any imbalance may give rise to blood disorders [1].

Myeloproliferative (the abnormal proliferation of myelopoietic cells that are present in the bone marrow) neoplasms (MPNs) are a group of blood disorders and cancer which occur after a somatic mutation in the cells of bone marrow. Following these mutations, the number of cells (RBCs, WBCs and platelets) produced in the bone marrow increase abnormally, eventually leading to diseases. MPNs are generally progressive disorders and they worsen over time. There are a number of treatment options and they can be applied either individually or in combination with another treatment option. In addition, new clinical trials have proven additional benefits to the patients.

According to World Health Organization's (WHO) 2016 list, the MPNs are classified as chronic myeloid leukemia (CML), chronic neutrophilic leukemia (CNL), polycythemia vera (PV), primary myelofibrosis (PMF), essential thrombocythemia (ET), chronic eosinophilic leukemia (CEL), and there is also unclassifiable MPNs (MPN-U). The majority of patients have only one type of MPNs, while some others may experience multiple types as the cells may be transformed to another type or into acute myeloid leukemia (AML) [2].

It is widely believed that genetic factors play a major role in development of MPNs. Most patients with MPNs have not reported a family history, which suggests that autosomal mutations are prominent in development of these disorders. However, a few familial cases have been reported, while it is quite difficult to distinguish the difference between sporadic and familial inheritance pattern within these cases. Due to accumulation of mutations, these neoplasms are more common in older people. These genetic defects mostly cause overproduction of one or more myeloid lineages such as granulocytic, megakaryocytic and erythroid lineages. The most prominent genes in MPNs include but are not limited to *JAK2*, *MPL*, *CALR*, *CSF3R*, *DNMT3A*, *TET2*, *SETBP1*, *RUNX1* [3, 4].

Hereditary forms of MPNs can be classified as two different groups. In the first group (Hereditary MPN-like disorders), there is polyclonal hematopoiesis, high penetrance with autosomal dominant inheritance and the single lineage is affected with Mendelian inheritance, and in the second group (True MPN disorders), the penetrance is incomplete with autosomal dominant inheritance. However, an autosomal recessive pattern has also been proposed [3]. Unlike solid tumors, MPNs do have clear anatomic features and the symptoms are similar. Therefore, it is necessary to use the diagnostic tools such as genetic testing, pathologic and histologic investigations all together to make a discrimination between the different types of MPNs. In order to diagnose the MPNs, a simple decision tree is used. Briefly, in *BCR-ABL1* (-) cases, one of the first things to consider is to investigate the *JAK2* V617F mutation in patients. If the patient is *JAK2* V617F (+), then diagnosis with PV, ET and PMF is likely. This leads to determine the subtypes of MPNs, based on the WHO criteria. If the patient is *JAK2* V617F (-), then mutations in *JAK2* exon 12, *CALR* and *MPL* genes must be investigated [5].

This chapter mainly focuses on the diagnostic criteria and molecular markers of the major myeloproliferative neoplasms, along with CML. In addition, the treatment options are briefly described.

PRIMARY MYELOFIBROSIS (PMF)
(AKA CHRONIC IDIOPATHIC MYELOFIBROSIS)

Primary myelofibrosis (PMF) is a rare disorder that occurs due to excessive accumulation of blood components and thick fibers in the bone marrow. It is usually a slow-progressing disorder that is diagnosed in 1.5/100,000 people and can be reversible, and the patient may spend years without even knowing that he/she has the disease. The median survival is between 1-5 years, while some patients may live longer [6]. However, myelofibrosis has a tendency to worsen over the time and can be lethal, if left untreated. Due to an acquired mutation in certain genes, the hematopoietic cells start to proliferate with an uncontrolled manner and immature cells (blasts) begin to form. These blasts are generally unable to function properly, and by the time, they block the bone marrow's ability to produce healthy blood cells, resulting in anemia in more than half of the patients. Patients with anemia often experience dyspnea (shortness of breath), fatigue, weakness, arrhythmia (irregular heart beat), cold extremities, and some others. When the bone marrow becomes defective, it also loses its ability to produce WBCs, which will eventually lead to decreased immune response and increased susceptibility to infections. In addition, the patients may experience bleeding problems and bruising due to decreased number of thrombocytes, whose main function is in formation of blood clots together with clotting proteins. If hematopoiesis is done out of the bone marrow in organs such as lungs, spleen, liver and spinal cord, this is called "medullary hematopoiesis", which may lead to splenomegaly (enlargement of the spleen) [7].

If the hematopoietic stem cells undergo a number of mutations, they may change the bone marrow to a fibrous structure. One of these cells that cause a change in bone marrow is the megakaryocytes, which have the ability of producing thrombocytes. Due to the mutations, the number of megakaryocytes increase in number which release cytokines, a special group of soluble proteins that are responsible for signaling between the cells, regulating immunity, hematopoiesis and inflammatory response. Since the number of megakaryocytes is more than necessary, the amount of cytokines is also increased that triggers formation of a thick fibrous tissue in the bone marrow, which will gradually destroy the healthy bone marrow [8].

Diagnosis of PMF

Since PMF is a slowly developing disorder, the patients may not be aware of the changes instantly. The diagnosis is usually coincidental. However, due to anemia, they may start to feel weakness, fatigue, and dyspnea, their liver may enlarge (hepatomegaly), due to low number of platelets (thrombocytopenia), they may bleed more frequently and easily, they may lose weight, excessive night sweats and fever are more pronounced, and they are more prone to infections because of low number of WBCs. If the patient has one or more complaints, the diagnosis can be made by physical exam, laboratory tests that will count blood cells and a bone marrow aspiration and biopsy may be required. If the patient has no symptoms but splenomegaly and abnormal laboratory results are present, it is plausible to think of "reactive myelofibrosis", which is a secondary reaction to an underlying problem such as an autoimmune disorder, chronic inflammatory conditions, leukemia, and infections [8].

A complete blood count can reveal anemia (low levels of RBCs), leukocytosis (high levels of WBCs), and leukopenia (low levels of WBCs). The platelet count is often abnormal. Using a peripheral blood smear test, the shape of the blood cells can be viewed under a microscope that will show the blasts (immature blood cells) and abnormally shaped (teardrop-shaped) RBCs. In addition, in order to have an idea about the organs' status, the physician may order a metabolic panel to investigate the levels of electrolytes (chloride, sodium, potassium), glucose, proteins and fats. Patients with PMF may have increased levels of lactic dehydrogenase (LDH-an enzyme that catalyzes the conversion of lactate to pyruvate, and high levels of LDH is an indicator of tissue damage and severity of the disease), uric acid (a natural metabolic waste product that forms after digestion of purines, high levels of uric acid (hyperurecemia) is an indicator of kidney failure, kidney stones, leukemia, PV, diabetes and some other problems and lower levels may be an indicator of Fanconi syndrome, liver disease, HIV infection, etc.), alkaline phosphatase (ALP-an enzyme in blood and high levels of ALP may show liver damage), and bilirubin (a protein that forms after break-down of RBCs and is an indicator of liver damage). However, it must be kept in mind that additional tests may be required as these alone may not be adequate for diagnosis. Bone marrow tests such as bone marrow aspiration and bone marrow biopsy to investigate the chromosomes may be necessary for a differential diagnosis and to discriminate PMF from other MPNs [9]. Scarring of the bone marrow (fibrosis) and the megakaryocytes with increased number and abnormal shapes can be detected by these methods. Ultrasonography (USG) and magnetic resonance imaging (MRI) techniques can be useful in detecting the changes in bone marrow. Human leukocyte antigen (HLA) typing is a method that investigates the cell surface receptors/proteins of the immune cells which are responsible for the regulation of the immune system. These proteins are encoded by the major histocompatibility complex (MHC) genes and HLAs are classified into three classes, namely MHC Class I, Class I and Class III, all with different functions in immune system. They can be used as a marker to determine whether the patients who need organ or stem cell transplantation will accept or reject the transplanted organ [10].

Molecular genetic methods can also be used for diagnostic purposes to determine the gene mutations that cause the diseases and by determining the type of the mutation, the treatment can be planned accordingly. WHO has included these molecular testing methods and they recommend to investigate *JAK2*, *CALR*, *MPL*, *TET2*, *ASXL1*, *BCR-ABL1* genes, and 13q deletions [6]. Approximately 90% of the patients with PMF are detected with either one of the *JAK2*, *CALR*, or *MPL* mutations. About 65-95% of the patients with PMF have *JAK2* V617F mutation [8, 11], 25% have *CALR* exon 9 deletions and insertions, 10% have *MPL* mutation, 17% have *TET2* mutation, 4%

have *IDH1/2* mutation, 13% have *ASXL1* mutation, 7% have *SF3B1* mutation, 13-17% have *SRSF2* mutation [8, 12], 16% have *U2AF1* mutation, and 7% have *DNMT3A* mutation [8]. Chromosomal abnormalities such as −7, inv(3), i(17q), +19, +21, del(12p), and del(11q), and various changes in chromosomes 3q21, 11q23 and 12p11.2 should also be investigated. In addition, total and partial trisomies (trisomy 1q, trisomy 8, trisomy 9, trisomy 9p, trisomy 13), del(5q), del(7q), del(13q), del(20q) have been reported in a number of cases with PMF [13, 14].

In 2016, WHO has announced that diagnosis of PMF should be based on three major criteria and one minor criterion. The major criteria are as follows:

Major criteria 1) Presence of fibrosis in bone marrow accompanied by abnormal megakaryocytes,

Major criteria 2) Presence of gene mutations (*JAK2, CALR, MPL, IDH1/2, ASXL1, EZH2, SF3B1, SRSF2, TET2*), and/or absence of reactive myelofibrosis, and,

Major criteria 3) Exclusion of PV, ET, *BCR-ABL1* (+) CML and other myeloid neoplasms and myelodysplastic syndromes (MDSs).

Minor criteria should include at least one of the followings:

WBC count ≥ 11×10^9/L, palpable splenomegaly, increased levels of LDH, presence of leukoerythroblastosis (immature blood cells in peripheral blood), anemia that is present due to another reason than any comorbid conditions. These should be found in consecutive two tests.

For treatment options, the patients are scored based on International Prognostic Scoring System (IPSS), or Dynamic International Prognostic Scoring System (DIPSS) (The scoring systems are based on age, WBC count, hemoglobin levels, blast ratio in peripheral blood, thrombocyte count, karyotyping, and constitutional symptoms) [15, 16]. The final score is used to assess the risk level from low to high. Primarily, diagnosis with triple negative mutations [*JAK2 (-), CALR (-)* and *MPL (-)*] has been associated with bad prognosis [5]. Based on the risk score and health status, the patients can be informed and under the guidance of an health professional, they can be directed to choose among a number of treatment options, such as allogeneic stem cell transplant, clinical trials, hydroxyurea (a DNA replication inhibitor), ruxolitinib (a JAK1 and JAK2 tyrosine kinases inhibitor), ganetespib (a heat shock protein inhibitor), vorinostat and givinostat (histone deacetylase inhibitors), everolimus (phosphatidylinositol-3'-kinase (PI3K), protein kinase B (AKT) and mechanistic target of rapamycin (mTOR) inhibitor), cytoreductive treatment, and splenectomy [6]. The advantages and disadvantages must be discussed thoroughly.

POLYCYTHEMIA (RUBRA) VERA (PV)

Polycythemia vera (PV) is a non-curable, but manageable rare disorder that is one of the myeloproliferative neoplasms. It is the most common MPN with an incidence of 0.6-1.6/million people in the USA. It can affect people at any age, but it is more frequent in elderly and rare in young children. The number of WBCs, RBCs and thrombocytes are elevated due to an acquired mutation in the stem cells of bone marrow. As the cells are mutated, the hematopoiesis is out-of-control, resulting in abnormal bleeding and clotting of blood, which will increase the risk of pulmonary embolism, heart attack, splenomegaly, and stroke [17].

PV is a slow-progressing disorder and the patient may live for years without any specific symptoms. Similar to PMF, the disorder is detected coincidentally during a physical exam or blood test. The symptoms may include fatigue, weakness, tinnitus (ringing in the ears), excessive sweating, increased production of sputum, wheezing, chronic cough, headaches, dyspnea (shortness of breath), impaired vision, pruritus (itching), numbness, weight loss, and inflammatory arthritis. Splenomegaly is detected in almost 3/4 of all patients with PV. However, as these symptoms may also be indicators of other diseases, other conditions should also be considered. Some patients may experience gout due to accumulation of uric acid in blood as uric acid is a by-product of shredded blood cells. As there are more blood cells, the level of uric acid can increase, causing pain and swelling of feet and toes. Some patients suffer from a burning, intense pain in hand and feet and episodic fevers. As the number of RBCs increases in blood circulation, organs with thin skin such as ear lobes, palms of the hands, soles of the feet and eyes may look reddish [17].

In certain cases, inherited diseases, high altitude, erythropoietin (EPO) secreting kidney or liver tumors, adrenal adenomas and diseases causing hypoxia may trigger "secondary polycythemia". Since this is not a cancer, it may arise due to above mentioned conditions and it can be treated by understanding and identifying the underlying cause.

Diagnosis of PV

In PV, patients are usually diagnosed with increased levels of RBCs, WBCs, platelets, hematocrit (ratio of RBC volume to the total blood volume) and hemoglobin. This can be easily measured by performing a complete blood count. Hematocrit levels greater than 48% in females and 52% in males, and hemoglobin levels greater than 16.5 g/dL in females and 18.5 g/dL in males are markers of PV [7, 8]. A peripheral blood smear can show the presence of blast cells and unusual changes in shape, size and appearance of the blood cells. A liquid bone marrow sample or bone marrow biopsy can help diagnose the PV, as abnormal changes in the number of megakaryocytes, the cells responsible for producing the platelets, will be detected in the tests. A comprehensive biochemical laboratory test can be used to detect the levels of erythropoietin, proteins, enzymes, fats, glucose and other chemical substances. Erythropoietin is a key hormone that is produced in kidneys and in liver in smaller amounts. It has a major function in production of red blood cells and the levels of EPO is very low in patients with PV because increased levels of hematocrit, hemoglobin, RBCs suppress the production of EPO. However, in secondary polycythemias, the levels of EPO can be normal or elevated and this information can be used to distinguish the primary and secondary polycythemias.

Molecular testing is a very useful tool in diagnosing PV. A positive *JAK2* V617F mutation and low levels of EPO is helpful in identifying PV. Approximately 90% of patients with PV have a positive *JAK2* V617F mutation [8]. In some cases, *JAK2* V617F mutation analysis can be negative and EPO levels are low. Then, analysis of exon 12 of the *JAK2* gene may be performed to diagnose PV. On the other hand, cytogenetic analysis can also help detect PV. Chromosomal abnormalities may be seen in approximately 14-40% of the patients with PV [18, 19]. Total or partial trisomies (trisomy 1q, trisomy 8, trisomy 9, trisomy 9p), del(5q), del(13q), del(20q), unbalanced translocations, loss of heterozygosity (LOH) of chromosome 9p have been reported in patients with PV [13]. Among these, del(20q), +8 and +9 are the most common abnormalities [19, 20].

In 2016, WHO has determined the major and minor criteria for diagnosing PV. In order to diagnose a patient with PV, the patient must either have three major criteria or two major and one minor criteria:

Major criteria 1) Presence of polycythemia (very high RBC count) accompanying either,

- (a) increased levels of hematocrit (>48% and 49% in women and men, respectively), or
- (b) increased levels of hemoglobin >16.0 g/dL and 16.5 g/dL in women and men, respectively), or
- (c) increased red cell mass.

Major criteria 2) Bone marrow biopsy either with,

- (a) presence of hypercellularity (excessive number of blood cells in bone marrow) together with increased number of RBCs, WBCs and thrombocytes (panmyelosis), or
- (b) increased number of mature megakaryocytes with abnormal shape.

Major criteria 3) *JAK2* V617F mutation or in some cases, *JAK2* exon 12 gene mutation.

Minor criterion: Decreased and very low levels of EPO (<4 mU/mL) [7].

For treatment options, if the risk is low, then phlebotomy (blood drawing process form veins) or low-dose aspirin can be started. If the risk is high, then cytoreductive treatment (depending on the stage, INF-α, hydoxyurea, busulphane/^{32}P) can be selected, low-dose aspirin, and phlebotomy can be performed, if necessary. Molecular response is not necessary to determine the complete or partial response. The measures for response to treatment are as follows:

Complete response: Complete response is the loss of previously present abnormality.

(a) Continuous improvement in symptoms and palpable hepatosplenomegaly, and,
(b) continuous response in peripheral blood count, hematocrit levels <45% without phlebotomy, platelet count <400x10^9/L, WBC count <10x10^9/L, and,
(c) absence of progressive disease symptoms and absence of hemorrhagic or thrombotic events,
(d) histologic response in bone marrow, presence of age-related normocellularity, loss of trilinear hyperplasia and absence of Grade 1 reticulin fibrosis.

Partial response: Partial response is defined as 50% decrease in allele load.

(a) Continuous improvement in symptoms and palpable hepatosplenomegaly, and,
(b) continuous response in peripheral blood count, hematocrit levels <45% without phlebotomy, platelet count <400x10^9/L, WBC count <10x10^9/L, and,
(c) absence of progressive disease symptoms and absence of hemorrhagic or thrombotic events,
(d) absence of histologic remission in bone marrow, persistence of trilinear hyperplasia.

No response: Any response that does not meet partial response.

Progressive disease: Post-PV myleofibrosis, transformation to AML or MDS [5].

About 96% of the patients with PV have *JAK2* V617F mutation, 3% have *JAK2* exon 12 mutation, 16% have *TET2* mutation, 2% have *IDH1/2* mutation, and 7% have *DNMT3A* mutation [8].

ESSENTIAL THROMBOCYTHEMIA (ET)

Essential thrombocythemia (ET) is a rare blood disorder that develops due to excessive number of thrombocytes in the blood. Due to an acquired mutation in DNA, the megakaryocytes are overproduced in bone marrow, and they increase in number causing release of excessive number of thrombocytes into the circulation [21]. Since the main function of thrombocytes is in blood clotting process, this may cause undesired formation of blood clots, and if left untreated, it may lead to serious health problems such as pulmonary embolism, heart attack, stroke, ischemia, and even death, due to blockage in large vessels and arteries. The disorder is called essential thrombocythemia because the patient is born with the disorder. On the other hand, the disorder may develop due to some other underlying conditions such as splenectomy, iron deficiency, and inflammatory diseases, and this is called "secondary or reactive thrombosis". If the underlying problem is solved, the patient may recover.

The symptoms of ET develop very slowly over the time and are similar to other MPNs. These can be listed as weakness, fatigue, chest pain, loss of vision, tinnitus, numbness and coldness in extremities due to blockage in small vessels, redness and pain in hands, feet and ears, deep vein thrombosis (DVT), and less likely, bleeding, easy bruising and bloody stool. ET is more common in elderly people, however, every person at any age can have the disorder. In some cases, ET may progress to other life-threatening conditions such as primary myelofibrosis and acute myeloid leukemia, even though the risk is about 1-2% for AML and 9% for PMF [21, 22].

Diagnosis of ET

The ET is usually diagnosed during a routine blood test or bone marrow sampling as the affected persons may not show the symptoms until advanced stages. A physical exam and blood tests along with other testing methods will help the doctor diagnose the patient with ET. In patients with ET, the platelet count is above average (>450,000/µL, for at least two months), the hemoglobin and hematocrit levels are also increased. Approximately 1/3 of patients with ET may have increased numbers of RBCs and/or WBCs. A peripheral blood smear can help identify the disorder if there are abnormally shaped blood cells and clustered or enlarged thrombocytes. A biochemistry laboratory test can reveal the changes in levels of proteins, fats, electrolytes (sodium, potassium, chloride), enzymes and glucose. Similar to other MPNs, a bone marrow biopsy or liquid bone marrow sample can help identify the shape, size and count of megakaryocytes. In addition, genetic testing for certain genes such as *JAK2*, *CALR* and *MPL* genes can help for a more accurate diagnosis [22, 23].

However, other diagnostic criteria must be considered to rule out other possibilities. In 2016, WHO announced the diagnostic criteria for ET. Based on this system, a patient must meet either four major criteria or three major criteria and one minor criterion in order to be diagnosed with ET [5].

Major criteria 1) The number of thrombocytes must be greater than 450,000/µL for a certain period of time,

Major criteria 2) Increased number of enlarged and mature megakaryocytes with hyperlobulated nuclei must be detected in bone marrow biopsy, there must not be any neutrophil granulopoiesis or erythropoiesis and riticulin fibers must be very low in number,

Major criteria 3) PMF, PV, *BCR-ABL1* (+) CML and other myelodysplastic syndromes and myeloid neoplasms must have been excluded,

Major criteria 4) Mutation in *JAK2*, *CALR* and *MPL* genes must be detected. *JAK2* and *MPL* gene mutations are detected almost in 50% and 10% of the patients with ET, respectively.

Minor criterion: A clonal marker must be present or reactive thrombocytosis must be detected.

For treatment options, if the risk is low, then low-dose aspirin can be started or the patient can be monitored. If the risk is high, then cytoreductive treatment (depending on the stage, INF-α, hydoxyurea, anagrelide can be selected) can be preferred. Molecular response is not necessary to determine the complete or partial response. The measures for response to treatment are as follows:

Complete response: Complete response is the loss of previously present abnormality.

(a) Continuous improvement in symptoms and palpable hepatosplenomegaly, and,
(b) continuous response in peripheral blood count, platelet count <400x10^9/L, WBC count <10x10^9/L, absence of leukoerythtoblastosis, and,
(c) absence of progressive disease symptoms and absence of hemorrhagic or thrombotic events, and,
(d) absence of histologic remission in bone marrow, loss of megakaryocyte hyperplasia, and absence of Grade 1 reticulin fibrosis.

Partial response: Partial response is defined as 50% decrease in allele load.

(a) Continuous improvement in symptoms and palpable hepatosplenomegaly, and,
(b) continuous response in peripheral blood count, hematocrit levels <45% without phlebotomy, platelet count <400x10^9/L, WBC count <10x10^9/L, and,
(c) absence of progressive disease symptoms and absence of hemorrhagic or thrombotic events,
(d) absence of histologic remission in bone marrow, persistence of megakaryocyte hyperplasia.

No response: Any response that does not meet partial response.

Progressive disease: Post-ET myelofibrosis, transformation to AML or MDS [5].

About 55% of the patients with ET have *JAK2* V617F mutation, 20% have *CALR* exon 9 deletion or insertion, 3% have *MPL* mutation, 5% have *TET2* mutation, 3% have *ASXL1* mutation, 1% have *IDH1/2* mutation, and 1% have various *RAS* mutations [8]. Chromosomal aberrations are not very frequent in patients with ET and the incidence is about 5-6% [18]. del(5q), del(20q), trisomies 8 and 9 are the reported chromosomal aberrations in patients with ET [13].

CHRONIC MYELOID (MYELOGENOUS) LEUKEMIA (CML)

Leukemia is a type of cancer that develops in bone marrow due to changes in the myeloid cells (hematopoietic stem cells) that are responsible for forming WBCs (except lymphocytes), RBCs and megakaryocytes. Basically, it is the cancer of WBCs and bone marrow. CML comprises about 1/4 of all leukemias and it can develop at any age but is more common in elderly and in males (M/F: 1.2/1 to 1.7) [24]. The prognosis is generally slow and the incidence is 1-2/100,000 cases. In CML, the number of granulocytes is greatly increased which do not function like healthy WBCs. In addition to granulocytes, the number of platelets may also increase in number. CML occurs due to genetic changes in the cell. A balanced reciprocal translocation between the 9th and 22nd chromosomes form a new chromosome called Philadelphia (Ph) chromosome t(9;22)(q34;q11), meaning that the *BCR* (Breakpoint Cluster Region) gene that is located on the 11q band of 22nd and *ABL1* (Abelson Murine Leukemia Viral Oncogene Homolog 1) gene that is located on the 34q band of 9th chromosome are joined together to form a fusion gene called *BCR-ABL1*. In addition, 5-10% of CML patients have variant Ph translocations which can be either simple or complex translocations. Simple variant translocations occur between chromosome 22 and any other chromosome than 9. In complex variant translocations 3 or more chromosomes are involved. Kuru et al. have demonstrated various variant Ph translocations such as t(7;22)(p22;q11), t(12;22)(p13;q11), t(15;22)(p11;q11), t(1;9;22;3)(q24;q34;q11;q21), t(9;22;15)(q34;q11;q22), t(4;8;9;22)(q11;q13;q34;q11) in patients with CML [25].

BCR-ABL1 is an oncogene and since *BCR* gene has three possible breakpoint regions, it may encode different hybrid proteins with different pathogenic effects. These breakpoints are called major *bcr* (M-*bcr*), minor *bcr* (m-*bcr*) and micro *bcr* (μ-*bcr*), and they give rise to different sized BCR-ABL1 fusion proteins, namely p210, p190 and p230, respectively [26]. The p210 is generally present in hematopoietic cells of patients with CML, and also in patients with ALL (Acute Lymphocytic Leukemia) and AML. p190 can be found in less than 5% of patients with CML, in addition, it is also present in Ph-positive [Ph (+)] acute B lymphoid leukemia and sometimes in AML [26, 27]. p230 is a less frequently detected fusion protein that was shown to be associated with AML, neutrophilic CML and classical CML [27, 28]. These proteins have tyrosine kinase activity that activates signaling molecules involved in JAK/STAT (Janus Kinase/Signal Transducers and Activators of Transcription), MAPK/ERK (Mitogen-activated Protein Kinase/Extracellular Signal-regulated Kinase), PI3K/AKT (Phosphatidylinositol-3′-Kinase/Protein Kinase B) signaling pathways, resulting in uncontrolled proliferation of the cells, hence cancer [29].

CML has three stages: chronic stage (85%), accelerated stage (10%), and blastic stage (5%) [30]. Since this is a slow-progressing disease and symptoms may not be detected on time, untreated patients advance to the blastic stage. This progression is usually accompanied with +8, +19, i(17q), and an extra Ph chromosome [31]. These patients are prone to heavy hemorrhages, anemia, infection, and multiple organ failure. Therefore, early diagnosis is of major importance to start the treatment as soon as possible. As *BCR-ABL1's* product is a tyrosine kinase, the treatment is usually given with tyrosine kinase inhibitors (TKIs) such as Imatinib to stop the uncontrolled proliferation of the cells.

Patients with CML show symptoms such as fatigue, weakness, weight loss, excessive night sweats, fever, bone pain, splenomegaly, fullness in abdomen, and some other symptoms.

Diagnosis of CML

Similar to other disorders, CML can share symptoms with other disorders. So, extensive physical examinations and laboratory tests must be performed to distinguish the disorders from each other. A physical examination will help detect whether the patient has an enlarged spleen but approximately 10% of all patients do not have it. A blood test can show that the number of leukocytes has increased to 100,000/mm^3 (the normal range is between 4,000-10,000/mm^3). In anemia and chronic phase, the thrombocyte count may have been elevated. Depending on the stage of the disorder, the number of thrombocytes can be either low or high. A peripheral blood smear test can be helpful in investigating the shape, count, ratio and any abnormalities of the blood cells. A few blast cells or promyelocytes, and more mature WBCs such as myelocytes and neutrophils can be detected under microscope. Bone marrow sampling and bone marrow liquid biopsy can be ordered to visualize the structure and number of chromosomes [30]. These chromosomal aberrations can be shown either with cytogenetic methods using G-banding and fluorescent *in situ* hybridization method (FISH), and molecular methods such as reverse transcription polymerase chain reaction (RT-PCR). In addition, the level of leukocyte alkaline phosphatase (LAP) which is low in patients with CML can be detected using cytochemical assays. A higher LAP score may be an indicator of ET, PV, PMF, and leukemoid reaction (increased number of WBCs due to an infection or stress), while a lower LAP score is common in CML, pernicious anemia, aplastic anemia, and AML [32].

The WHO has published the latest criteria for diagnosis of CML [2].

Complete hematologic response (CHR): A complete hematologic response is defined as when a patient with CML has normal blood values, there are no immature cells and their size and shape is normal, and there is no splenomegaly.

- The WBC count should be <10,000/µL,
- Absence of myeloblasts, promyelocytes and myelocytes in peripheral blood,
- Basophil count should be <5%,
- Thrombocyte count <450,000/µL
- No palpable splenomegaly.

Partial hematologic response (PHR): If the blood counts have improved but the patient still shows symptoms of CML, then he/she has a PHR. WBC count has reduced to half compared to the day 1 of the treatment, the number of thrombocytes is still above average, and even though the spleen has reduced in size, it is still palpable.

Cytogenetic response (CyR): A cytogenetic response is when the patient with CML has no Ph chromosome in at least 20 cells in metaphase plaque which were obtained from a bone marrow sample. The cytogenetic response can be classified in different groups:

- No Ph (+) metaphase,
- Partial cytogenetic response (PCyR) should be Ph (+) metaphase 1-35% (up to 35% of all cells have a Ph chromosome),
- Minor cytogenetic response should be Ph (+) metaphase 36-65% (36-65% of all cells have a Ph chromosome),
- Minimal cytogenetic response should be Ph (+) metaphase 66-95% (66-95% of all cells have a Ph chromosome),
- No cytogenetic response means >95% of all cells still have Ph chromosome.

If the cytogenetic response is based on FISH analysis, then false positivity rate of the laboratory should also be considered.

Molecular response (MR): The molecular response is based on the results obtained from polymerase chain reaction (PCR) tests. Presence and/or copy number of the gene determines the level of molecular response.

Complete molecular response (CMR): There are no copies of *BCR-ABL1* gene in blood.

Major molecular response (MMR, MR 3.0 or deeper response): The *BCR-ABL1/ABL1* ratio is ≤0.1%.

MR 4.0 is as follows:

(a) Detectable molecular disease, *BCR-ABL1* copy number is <0.01%,
(b) Undetectable molecular disease, >10,000 copies of *ABL1*.

MR 4.5 is as follows:

(a) Detectable molecular disease, *BCR-ABL1* copy number is <0.0032%,
(b) Undetectable molecular disease, >32,000 copies of *ABL1* [2, 33].

Follow-Up of Treatment Response

The hematologic evaluation is performed every 15 days until a complete hematologic response is achieved, and then every 3 months or whenever it is necessary. The cytogenetic evaluation is made at baseline, at months 3 and 6, every 6 months until a complete cytogenetic response is achieved, and then every 12 months after complete cytogenetic response. If there is no response to treatment (primary or secondary resistance), and if there is leukopenia, thrombocytopenia and anemia, the cytogenetic evaluation should be performed continuously.

A number of drugs can be prescribed to treat the patients with CML. Tyrosine kinase inhibitors (TKIs) are the first drug of choice and Imanitinib is generally selected as a first-line treatment. In this context, the responses are classified as optimal response, warning and no-response. For the optimal response, at baseline, there is no available response. At month 3, the optimal response is defined as *BCR-ABL1* ≤%10 and/or Ph (+) ≤35%; at month 6, *BCR-ABL1* <1% and/or Ph (+) 0; at month 12 and at any time afterwards, *BCR-ABL1* ≤0.1%. For the warning response, at baseline, high risk or CCA/Ph (+), major route; at month 3, *BCR-ABL1* >10% and/or Ph (+) 36-95%; at month 6, *BCR-ABL1* 1-10% and/or Ph (+) 1-35%; at month 12, *BCR-ABL1* >0.1-1%; then, at any time, CCA/Ph (−) (−7, or 7q−). The no-response is classified as: at baseline, nothing; at month 3, non-CHR and/or Ph (+) >95%; at month 6, *BCR-ABL1* >10% and/or Ph (+) >35%; at month 12, *BCR-ABL1* >1% and/or Ph (+) >0; and, at any time, loss of CHR, loss of CCyR, confirmed loss of MMR, mutations, and CCA/Ph (+) (clonal chromosomal abnormalities) [33].

In case of failure or resistance to Imatinib, second-line tyrosine kinase inhibitors such as Nilotinib, Dasatinib, Bosutinib, Ponatinib can be started. For the optimal response, at baseline, there is no specific response. At month 3, the optimal response is defined as *BCR-ABL1* ≤%10 and/or Ph (+) ≤65%; at month 6, *BCR-ABL1* ≤%10 and/or Ph (+) <35%; at month 12, *BCR-ABL1* <1% and/or Ph (+) 0, then, at any time *BCR-ABL1* ≤0.1%. For the warning response, at baseline, no CHR or loss of CHR on imatinib or lack of CyR to first-line TKI or high risk; at month 3, *BCR-ABL1* >10% and/or Ph (+) 65-95%; at month 6, Ph (+)

35-65%; at month 12, *BCR-ABL1* 1-10% and/or Ph (+) 1-35%; and then, at any time, CCA/Ph (–) (–7 or 7q–) or *BCR-ABL1* >0.1%. The failure is classified as: at baseline, not available; at month 3, no CHR or Ph+ >95% or presence of new mutations; at month 6, *BCR-ABL1* >10% and/or Ph (+) >65% and/or new mutations, at month 12, *BCR-ABL1* >10% and/or Ph (+) >35% and/or new mutations, and then, at any time, loss of CHR or loss of CCyR or PCyR, new mutations, confirmed loss of MMR CCA/Ph (+) [33].

Based on the patient's status, the physician can plan the treatment options. The molecular response of the patients can be followed up using Sanger DNA sequencing or RT-PCR. A number of mutations of *BCR-ABL1* gene such as D276G, E255K, E255V, E279K, F311L, F317L, F317V, F359V, F486S, G250E, H396P, H396R, L248V, L384M, L387M, M244V, M351T, Q252H, T315I, T315A, V299L, V379I, Y253F, Y253H have been shown to be effective in changing the prognosis [33].

The mechanism of resistance to Imatinib has been a topic of debate. The point mutations around the phosphate-binding loop (P loop; positions M244, G250, Q252, Y253, and E255), gatekeeper residue (T315 and F317), SH2 contact and C-lobe (M351, F359), and the activation loop (H396) of the BCR-ABL1 protein has been preventing the binding of Imatinib, thus reducing the efficacy of treatment. On the other hand, some of these mutations can also be the reason of resistance to second-line treatment drugs such as Bosutinib, Nilatinib, Dasatinib. T315I mutation, which is called a gatekeeper mutation as it has an ATP binding site, can cause resistance to previously mentioned drugs [34]. On the other hand, resistance to treatment can develop based on mechanisms regardless of kinase mutations. Body of evidence has shown that signaling pathways including PI3K/AKT, JAK/STAT can also be the cause of resistance [35, 36]. Nevertheless, microenvironmental factors may also play a role in TKIs resistance [29].

CHRONIC EOSINOPHILIC LEUKEMIA, NOT OTHERWISE SPECIFIED (CEL NOS)

Chronic eosinophilic leukemia (CEL) is another rare MPN that develops due to excessive production of eosinophils in the bone marrow. Eosinophils are members of WBCs and are increased in number in case of an allergic reaction, parasitic and fungal infection, exposure to toxins, autoimmune and endocrine disorders, and cancer. Eosinophilia (increased number of eosinophils in blood, the normal count for eosinophils is usually less than 500 eosinophils/µL. 500-1,500 eosinophils/µL show mild, 1,500-5,000 eosinophils/µL show moderate and greater than 5,000 eosinophils/µL show severe eosinophilia) [37, 38] may occur due to a number of diseases and conditions other than CEL such as Hodgkin's lymphoma, asthma, allergy, Churg-Strauss syndrome, immunodeficiencies, ulcerative colitis, etc. Patients with CEL have a median survival of 22 months, and it is common to see that CEL can transform to acute leukemia [39].

Patients with CEL may show symptoms such as diarrhea, cough, fever, fatigue, angioedema, myalgia, and arthralgia because of elevated levels of cytokines from eosinophils. Since the eosinophils can accumulate in peripheral blood and tissues, they can be detected in skin, lungs, gastrointestinal tract, muscles and mucosal tissues. About 20% of the patients with CEL have cardiovascular symptoms and 50% have respiratory symptoms [40]. Patients can exhibit signs of splenomegaly and hepatomegaly. A number of patients can experience visual disturbances due to retinal thrombosis. Similar to other MPNs, the prognosis of CEL is due to genetic changes and it has an aggressive prognosis. CEL is classified as a *BCR-ABL1* (-) myeloproliferative neoplasm and can be diagnosed with *JAK2* fusion genes and absence of *FGFR1* (Fibroblast Growth Factor Receptor 1), *PDGFRA* (Platelet Derived Growth Factor Receptor A), and *PDGFRB* (Platelet Derived Growth Factor Receptor B) [41].

Diagnosis of CEL

CEL can be diagnosed with a number of methods. A complete blood count, blood chemistry tests and bone marrow aspiration and bone marrow biopsy are common ways of diagnosing patients with CEL. A complete blood count can show that patients with severe and persistent eosinophilia have an increased count of eosinophils ≥1.5x10^9/L (hypereosinophilia). The number of leukocytes is detected between 20,000-30,000. The count for blast cells should be ≥5%-<20% in bone marrow and ≥2%-<20% in peripheral blood and many mature eosinophils and only a few eosinophilic promyelocytes or myelocytes are also detected. inv(16)(p13;q22), t(16;16)(p13;q22), t(8;21)(q22;q22), and other diagnostic features of AML should not be present. t(5;12)(q31-35;p13) should be absent. Thrombocytopenia and anemia have been reported. A number of mutated genes such as *ASXL1*, *EZH2*, *JAK2*, *CBL*, *NOTCH1*, *DNMT3A* and *TET2* have been discovered in patients with CEL. The patients are diagnosed with CEL if the criteria for WHO for a *BCR-ABL1* (+) CML, atypical CML, ET, CMML (Chronic Myelomonocytic Leukemia), CNL, PV, PMF are not met. On the other hand, there should be no rearrangement of *PDGFRA*, *PDGFRB* or *FGFR1*, and no *PCM1-JAK2*, *ETV6-JAK2* or *BCR-JAK2* fusion genes. Since *FIP1L1-PDGFRA* rearrangement is very common in patients with CEL, molecular testing should be repeated in every three months in patients [42]. 100 mg of Imatinib treatment can be started in patients with *FIP1L1-PDGFRA* (+) CEL [43]. However, some patients may be resistant to Imatinib treatment due to T674I and D842V mutations in *FIP1L1-PDGFRA* gene [44].

UNCLASSIFIABLE MYELOPROLIFERATIVE NEOPLASMS (MPN-U)

A number of methods and tools have been used widely to disentangle the differences between common types of MPNs, while it is still a matter of debate if there is still unclassifiable MPN (MPN-U) [4, 45]. In fact, MPN-U constitute a large group of MDS/MPN categories

[46]. According to 2017 WHO classification, this category includes MDS/MPN with ring sideroblasts and thrombocytosis (MDS/MPN-RS-T), atypical chronic myeloid leukemia (aCML), chronic myelomonocytic leukemia (CMML), and MDS/MPN unclassifiable (MDS/MPN-U) [47].

Similar to other MPNs, the patients with MPN-U may experience excessive night sweats, cough, splenomegaly and weight loss. In addition, the level of thrombocytes and LDH can be elevated, while the levels of hemoglobin and WBCs can fall within the normal range [48]. In order for a patient to be diagnosed with MPN-U, the patients should not have a *BCR-ABL1* mutation and there should be no monocytosis, dysgranulopoiesis or dyserythropoiesis. In addition, erythrocytosis, thrombocytosis and peripheral blood granulocytosis should be detected. A recent study conducted in patients with MPN-U has shown *CALR* and *JAK2* V617F mutations in 37.5% and 25% of the patients, respectively, while the remaining 37.5% had no mutations in *JAK2*, *CALR* or *MPL* genes (triple negative) [49]. In another study, more than 70% of the patients with MPN-U had a *JAK2* V617F mutation and of the *JAK2* (-) patients, 17% and 67% of the patients had *MPL* W515L and *CALR* gene mutations (del52bp, ins5bp, del46 bp, del2bp in exon 9), respectively [48]. Another study has shown that *ZBTB33* gene is mutated in patients with MDS/MPN-U [4]. However, these mutations do not make a great contribution to diagnosis of MPN-U, as they do in other types of MPNs [50].

On the other hand, other subtypes of MDS/MPNs show a heterogeneous distribution for molecular genetic changes. For example, approximately half of the patients with CMML harbor *TET2*, *SRSF2*, *ASXL1* mutations and *TET2-SRSF2* fusion [51]. *ASXL1*, *TET2*, *NRAS*, *SETBP1*, and *RUNX1 gene mutations are detected in patients with aCML [52, 53], and about 90% of the patients with* MDS/MPN-RS-T are carriers of *SF3B1* gene mutation, along with *JAK2* V617F mutation [54]. Mutations of *TET2*, *DNMT3A*, and *ASXL1* have also been detected in MDS/MPN-RS-T [55].

MOLECULAR CHANGES IN PHILADELPHIA CHROMOSOME-NEGATIVE [PH (-)] MPNS

In addition to the chromosomal aberrations mentioned above, a number of somatic mutations have been documented in Ph (-) MPNs such as PV, ET, PMF and CNL, which affect the prognosis of the patients. Therefore, it is of major importance to investigate and understand the effects of these genetic changes to develop new treatment strategies. The major genes involved in Ph (-) MPNs development are *JAK2*, *MPL*, *CALR*, *CSF3R*, and their mutations are called the driver mutations. On the other hand, there are passenger mutations in other genes such as *DNMT3A*, *TET2*, *IDH1*, *IDH2*, *ASXL1*, *EZH2*, *SRSF2*, *U2AF1*, *SF3B1* and *RUNX1* which accompany driver mutations.

Driver Mutations in Ph (-) MPNs

Driver mutations are genetic alterations that may occur in *JAK2*, *MPL*, *CALR*, *CSF3R* genes and directly lead to hyperproliferation of hematopoietic cells [11]. JAK2 V617F mutation is the first described gene mutation and the most frequently occurring somatic mutation in Ph (-) MPNs [56, 57].

JAK2 (Janus Kinase 2)

JAK2 (Janus Kinase 2) (OMIM, *147796) is a gene that is located on chromosome 9p24.1. The product of this gene is JAK2, one of the members of the Janus Kinase (JAK) family. This protein family comprises JAK1, JAK2, JAK3 and TYK2 that play an essential role in signal transduction from activated cytokine receptors into the cell. Upon ligand binding to cytokine receptors, JAKs are activated by transphosphorylation. Activated JAKs lead to phosphorylation of downstream adaptor and effector proteins including the signal transducers and activators of transcription (STAT) proteins. When phosphorylated, STAT family members (STAT1, STAT2, STAT3, STAT4, STAT5A, STAT5B and STAT6) are activated and translocate into the nucleus where they promote transcription of various cytokine-responsive genes [58, 59].

All members of the JAK family have common structural domains, namely N-terminal band 4.1, ezrin, radixin, moesin (FERM) domain and a Src homology 2 (SH2) domain, catalytically-defective pseudokinase (Jak homology 2, JH2) domain and enzymatically active C-terminal tyrosine kinase (Jak homology 1, JH1) domain. FERM and SH2 domains mediate the interaction between JAKs and the intracellular domain of cytokine receptors. JH1 domain has a kinase activity, while JH2 domain acts as a negative regulator of JH1 domain by inhibiting its catalytic activity [58, 60-62].

Activating mutations in JAKs play a central role in molecular pathogenesis of Ph (-) MPNs. The majority of these somatic mutations occur in the gene region encoding JH2 domain of the JAKs, resulting in constitutively active kinases [58]. Being the most frequent occurring somatic mutation, *JAK2* V617F frequency is around 65-95% in PV and 50-65% in ET and PMF [8, 11]. This missense mutation occurs in exon 14 of the *JAK2* gene (G to T exchange at nucleotide 1849) and causes a substitution of valine with phenylalanine at amino acid position 617 (V617F) within the JH2 domain resulting in increased tyrosine kinase activity of JAK2. Other than *JAK2* V617F mutation, somatic gain-of-function mutations have been detected in exon 12 of *JAK2* in patients with PV [63].

MPL (Myeloproliferative Leukemia Virus Oncogene)

The *MPL* (Myeloproliferative Leukemia Virus Oncogene) gene (OMIM, *159530), located on chromosome 1p34.2, encodes the thrombopoietin (TPO) receptor that regulates megakaryopoiesis and hematopoietic stem cell renewal, quiescence, and expansion [64, 65]. This single-pass membrane receptor contains a large extracellular domain, a single transmembrane domain, and an intracellular cytoplasmic domain. Binding of the ligand to the extracellular domain of the TPO receptor triggers formation of receptor dimers or the preformed dimers are structurally rearranged that changes rotational direction and/or association of the transmembrane helix and juxtamembrane regions of the receptor, so the receptor becomes active [66]. Receptor dimerization promotes cross-phosphorylation and activation of the tyrosine kinases JAK2 and TYK2. Activated JAKs then phosphorylate tyrosine residues in the TPO receptor intracellular domain that serve as docking platforms for downstream signaling molecules such as STAT3, STAT5, Src homologous and collagen (Shc), GRB2 (Growth Factor Receptor–Bound Protein 2), and PI3K which are involved in signal transduction [64, 67].

Single amino acid substitution by asparagine (N) in the transmembrane domain and cysteine (C) in the extracellular domain, and mutations in the intracellular and extracellular juxtamembrane domains of the TPO receptor result in ligand-independent dimerization and activation of the receptor [64]. Especially, missense mutations in *MPL* causing a change from tryptophan (W) to leucine (L), lysine (K), or alanine (A) at amino acid position 515 (*MPL* W515) are somatic activating mutations that occur in ET and PMF. As a consequence of these mutations, the inhibitor effect of the tryptophan residue at position 515 in the intracellular juxtamembrane domain on dimerization of the receptor is lost and the receptor becomes active [37, 67, 68]. Therefore, JAK/STAT signaling pathway is activated in a ligand-independent manner. The frequency of *MPL* W515 gain-of-function mutations is approximately 3-10% in ET and PMF, respectively, while they are absent in PV [8, 65]. Y252H and F126fs gain-of-function mutations are other reported *MPL* gene mutations that occur in patients with ET [69].

CALR (Calreticulin)

The *CALR* (Calreticulin) gene (also known as *CRT*, OMIM, *109091), located on chromosome 19p13.13, has 9 exons and encodes a 47kDa endoplasmic reticulum (ER) chaperone protein [70]. This multifunctional protein is predominantly found in the lumen of ER and in the cytoplasm. It is also localized in the nucleus and on the cell surface. Within the ER, the protein plays an essential role in folding of newly synthesized glycoproteins, interacts with other chaperones and regulates calcium homeostasis. Outside of the ER, calreticulin is involved in cell proliferation, cell migration, adhesion, apoptosis, and immunogenic cell death [70-72]. It also regulates transcriptional activity, and interacts with integrins, major actors of cell adhesion [70, 72].

Calreticulin is composed of 417 amino acids. This highly conserved protein has an amino acid signal sequence at the N-terminal (residues 1-17), three specialized functional domains (N-, P- and C- domains, respectively), and a KDEL (Lys-Asp-Glu-Leu) signal sequence at the C-terminal for preventing the secretion of proteins from ER and retrieval of misfolded proteins to ER. The N-terminal domain (residues 18-197) has a globular structure with chaperone function. It also binds Zn^{+2} and interacts with other ER chaperones and DNA-binding domain of nuclear receptors *in vitro*. The P-domain (residues 198-308) has a proline-rich sequence and it can interact with integrins via its lectin-like site and with Ca^{+2} via its calcium binding site. The C-terminal domain (residues 308-417) is rich in acidic amino acids and binds Ca^{+2} with high capacity. It also enables calreticulin to interact with other chaperones [70, 73]. N-terminal amino acid signal sequence (residues 1-17) and C-terminal KDEL signal sequence (residues 414-417) serve targeting and retention of calreticulin in the ER [70, 74]. The N- and P-domains also host six putative ubiquitination and nine putative acetylation sites, along with 14 putative JAK2 dependent phosphorylation sites that enable the protein to change its function [73].

More than 50 mutations in *CALR* gene have been reported in 70% to 80% of patients with ET and PMF with nonmutated *JAK2* and *MPL* genes. All these mutations occur in exon 9 of the *CALR* gene and consist of insertions and/or deletions. The most common two mutations of *CALR* are 52-base deletion (type 1: c.1092_1143del, (p.L367fs*46), shortly: del52) and 5-base insertion (type 2: c.1154_1155insTTGTC, (p.K385fs*47), shortly: ins5) mutations, which make up more than 80% of all *CALR* mutations [75]. All *CALR* mutations have been shown to cause frameshifts that change the reading frame, resulting in loss of the KDEL motif and generation of a novel C-terminal domain with positively charged amino acid sequence. The mutant CALR protein interacts with the TPO receptor MPL through its N-domain with N-glycan property (with substituted amino acids (D135L/Y109F)) and activates signaling molecules such as ERK1/2, STATs and AKT via JAK2, thus causing constitutive proliferation of the cell, and clonal expansion of hematopoietic stem cells [23, 75-78]. It has also been noted that *CALR* mutation carriers had a longer overall survival and reduced risk of thrombosis compared to those with mutated *JAK2* [75]. In addition to its prominent role in Ph (-) MPNs, *CALR* has been shown to play important roles in other types of solid cancers such as breast, ovarian, gastric, oral and esophageal squamous cell carcinomas [73].

CSF3R (Colony-Stimulating Factor 3 Receptor, Granulocyte)

The *CSF3R* (Colony-Stimulating Factor 3 Receptor, Granulocyte) gene (also known as *GCSFR* (Granulocyte Colony-Stimulating Factor (G-CSF) Receptor), OMIM, *138971), located on chromosome 1p34.3, encodes the transmembrane receptor for G-CSF. This receptor is a member of the hematopoietin receptor superfamily and plays a key role in proliferation, differentiation and survival of granulocytes. It also functions in cell surface adhesion [79-81].

CSF3R, consisting of 813 amino acids, has an extracellular ligand-binding domain, a transmembrane domain and a cytoplasmic domain. G-CSF binding to the extracellular domain of CSF3R triggers dimerization and activation of the receptor which induce JAK/STAT and PI3K/AKT signaling pathways [80, 82]. Activating missense mutations in exon 14 of *CSF3R* gene have been detected in 80% of patients with CNL. These mutations affect the extracellular domain of the receptor resulting ligand-independent activation of the JAK/STAT and PI3K/AKT signaling pathways. The most common *CSF3R* mutation in CNL is T618I mutation (sometimes annotated as T595I), being the diagnostic marker for CNL [80, 82, 83].

Passenger Mutations in MPNs

Passenger mutations are mutations that do not directly cause myeloproliferation, but can change the effect of the driver mutations.

Opposed to driver mutations, these mutations alone do not cause MPN disease initiation but they play role in disease progression if they accompany driver mutations. Passenger mutations can occur in genes that encode epigenetic regulators, transcription factors, or signaling molecules [11]. The most frequently mutated genes in MPNs are *TET2*, *DNMT3A*, *ASXL1*, and *EZH2*, whose products function as epigenetic regulators. Mutation in other genes are at lower frequencies [84, 85].

DNA Methylation Modifiers (*DNMT3A, TET2, IDH1* and *IDH2*)

Epigenetic modification of DNA is an important process in cell survival, genomic imprinting, hematopoietic stem cell differentiation, embryonic development, and X-chromosome inactivation. These modifications can change the function of DNA without changing its nucleotide sequence. A number of DNA methylation modifiers such as *DNMT3A*, *TET2*, *IDH1* and *IDH2* have been described in MPNs [86].

DNMT3A (DNA Methyltransferase 3 Alpha)

A methyltransferase is an enzyme which catalyzes transfer of a methyl group to the cytosine and guanine rich regions (CpG islands mainly found in promoters of genes). *DNMT3A* (DNA Methyltransferase 3 Alpha, OMIM, *602769) gene, located on chromosome 2p23.3, is responsible for encoding a 130 kDa methyltransferase that is required for de novo methylation. DNMT3A has three domains that are used to interact with DNA and other proteins. These are PWWP (Pro-Trp-Trp-Pro) domain, ADD domain (ATRX-DNMT3-DNMT3L), and the catalytic methyltransferase domain. The PWWP and ADD domains are regulatory domains, whereas the catalytic domain is involved in DNA methylation [87].

Mutation of *DNMT3A* has been described in patients with AML, where arginine 882 (R882) mutation within the C-terminal catalytic domain was the most frequently detected mutation with a ratio up to 22%. Nevertheless, other mutations such as frameshift, nonsense, splice-site mutations and a large deletion have been described in patients with AML [88]. Normally, the wild-type *DNMT3A* is hypermethylated, but a mutation in this R882 hotspot may cause the gene to be hypomethylated, thus reducing its methyltransferase activity [87]. Additionally, mutation of *DNMT3A* has been shown in 16% of patients with ET, and 15% of patients with PMF [86].

TET2 (Tet Methylcytosine Dioxygenase 2)

TET2 is a dioxygenase that plays active role in DNA demethylation by catalyzing the conversion of 5-methylcytosine (5mC) into 5-hydroxymethylcytosine (5hmC) by transferring an oxygen molecule to a methyl group. This protein is encoded by *TET2* (TET Methylcytosine Dioxygenase 2, or TET Oncogene Family, Member 2, OMIM, *612839) which is localized on 4q24 chromosomal region.

TET2 is an evolutionary conserved dioxygenase and a member of TET family that is composed of three TETs (TET1, TET2, and TET3). The TET proteins have a conserved CXXC-type zinc finger domain at amino terminal which is responsible for DNA binding. TET2 is abundantly expressed in neuronal and hematopoietic cells [89]. TET2 has a functional domain at C-end of the protein with a double-stranded β-helix fold (DSβH) domain and a cysteine-rich domain. The DSβH domain can bind iron and α-ketoglutarate. TET2 can interact with O-linked β-D-N-acetylglucosamine (O-GlcNAc) transferase (OGT) to add it to the chromatin structure, just to regulate the transcription by increasing H3K4me3 level. If the TET2 protein is truncated or the catalytic domain undergoes a mutation, the iron and ketoglutarate binding function is affected, thus causing DNA hypermethylation and impaired 5mC oxidation [90].

TET2 is an important actor in hematopoiesis and a deleterious mutation of *TET2* have been shown to affect stem/progenitor cell differentiation by increasing the ratio of immature c-Kit+Lin− cells [91]. *TET2* also acts a tumor suppressor gene and its loss-of-function has been associated with hematopoietic malignancies by causing myeloid lineage expansion and increased HSC self-renewal [90]. A variety of mutations including frame shifts, nonsense mutations, amino acid substitutions, and in frame deletions have been reported in 20-35% of patients with MDS, in 30-60% of patients with CMML, 12–34% in AML, and 2–33% in other lymphoid malignancies [92].

There is conflicting reports on the effect of *TET2* mutations on the overall survival (OS) of patients. Some studies have reported that mutations do not have significant effect on OS, while others have reported shorter survival, some have reported longer survival. A *TET2* mutation has been shown to induce AML with a co-existent *FLT3-ITD* mutation [93], while a mutated *TET2* with *ASXL1* and *JAK2* gene mutations caused development of PMF and PV [94, 95]. TET2 can also induce myelopoiesis by suppressing mRNA of Socs3, a negative regulator of JAK/STAT pathway [96]. It is plausible to think that the treatment options should concentrate on restoring the TET2 function in patients with MDS or hematopoietic problems.

IDH1 and *IDH2* (Isocitrate Dehydrogenase 1 and 2)

Isocitrate dehydrogenase 1 and 2 (IDH1 and IDH2) are members of isocitrate dehydrogenase family that consists five members (the others being IDH3, IDH4 and IDH5) and they are mostly found in the cytosol as dimers and their function is NAD and NADP dependent. These enzymes are functional in decarboxylation of isocitrate into alpha-ketoglutarate (or 2-oxoglutarate, a key player in Krebs cycle and amino acid production) and they are important in cellular processes such as DNA repair, redox reactions, and epigenetic regulation. IDH1 is located in the cytosol and is encoded by *IDH1* gene (OMIM, *147700), located on chromosome 2q34. On the other hand, IDH2 is found in the mitochondria and is encoded by *IDH2* gene (OMIM, *147650), located on chromosome 15q26.1.

IDH1 has two hydrophilic active sites and three domains. A large domain (residues 1-103 and 286-414), a small domain (residues 104-136 and 186-285) and a clasp domain (residues 137-185) [97]. Mutations of *IDH1* and *IDH2* have been implemented in a number of diseases including >80% of low-grade gliomas and secondary gliomas, 60% of chondrosarcomas and 10% of AML. The most common mutations occur in the active site of the protein and are R132H and

R132C (substituting arginine with histidine or cysteine, respectively) in *IDH1* and R140Q and R172K (substituting arginine with glutamine and lysine, respectively) in *IDH2* [98]. These missense mutations cause the NADPH to reduce αKG to D-2-hydroxyglutarate, which would inhibit histone demethylation, leaving the cell in a hypermethylated state, thus resulting in stopping the differentiation process of non-transformed cells and triggering over-proliferation of immature blood cells [99].

Chromatin Modifiers (*ASXL1, EZH2*)

ASXL1 (Additional Sex Comb Like-1)

ASXL1 (Additional Sex Comb Like-1) protein is the human homolog of asx gene in *Drosophila melanogaster*. This protein is a member of Polycomb proteins and is encoded by *ASXL1* gene (OMIM, *612990), located on chromosome 20q11.21 in humans. It has three domains: an N-terminus ASXN domain, an ASX homology (ASXH) domain at N-terminus, and a plant homeodomain (PHD) finger at C-terminus. The ASXN domain is functional in DNA binding and PHD domain is a histone or DNA binder [100]. ASXL1 is functional in chromatin remodeling, hence DNA packaging. This is an important process for controlling the gene expression. It silences developmental genes known as *HOX* (Homeobox) genes, and also helps regulate gene expression by mediating the methylation process through polycomb repressor complex 2 (PRC2), a member of polycomb-group proteins with histone methyltransferase activity. The mutations of *ASXL1* gene have been found to be associated with MPNs (34.5% in PMF, and rare in ET and PV, 6.5% in de novo AML cases and 34.5% in secondary AML cases, 45% in CMML, and in MDS (2nd most frequent mutated gene after *TET2*)). In addition, *ASXL1* mutations co-exist with other mutations such as *GATA2*, *RUNX1*, *EZH2*, *JAK2*, *RAS*, *U2AF1*, *U2AF35*, *DNMT3A* [95, 100]. *ASXL1* mutations are generally either frameshift or nonsense mutations and usually tend to occur at 5' end of exon 12, resulting in formation of a truncated protein [101]. A*SXL1* mutations are either loss- or gain-of function mutations. A loss-of-function of *ASXL1* is due to loss of PRC2 mediated histone H3 lysine 27 (H3K27) tri-methylation, which results in impaired repression of

HOXA gene [102], and a gain-of-function occurs if the ASXL1-BAP deubiqutinase complex is activated, which results in loss of H2K119 ubiqutination [103]. The most frequent mutation of *ASXL1* is duplication of a guanine nucleotide (c.1934dupG) that occurs almost in half of all *ASXL1* mutations and this mutation causes a frameshift mutation (p.Gly646TrpfsX12) [95].

EZH2 (Enhancer of Zeste 2 Polycomb Repressive Complex 2 Subunit)

EZH2 (Enhancer of Zeste 2 Polycomb Repressive Complex 2 Subunit) is another chromatin modifier protein, a catalytic component of PRC2, that transfers methyl groups to nucleosomal histone H3 at lysine K27 (H3K27), resulting in histone methylation and transcriptional repression. As in ASXL1, this methylation helps regulate the heterochromatin remodeling and DNA packaging. H3K27 can be mono-, di-, and trimethylated and regulates the expression activity of the target gene [104].

The protein is encoded by *EZH2* gene (OMIM, *601573), located on chromosome 7q36.1, and has three domains. The SET domain is at C-terminus and is responsible for methyl transferase activity, the ncRBD and CXC domains are functional in interacting with other regulatory proteins and PRC2 components [104]. *EZH2* has been shown to be overexpressed in a number of cancer types including lung, breast, ovarian, hepatocellular and prostate. In addition, *EZH2* gene overexpression and loss-of-function mutations have been detected in MDS. EZH2 can increase epithelial to mesenchymal transition (EMT) by down-regulating the E-cadherin and interacting with SNAIL [105, 106]. EZH2 also has functions in drug resistance to cancer treatment, tumor suppression, transcriptional and post-transcriptional regulation [104]. It has been shown that 6-13% of patients with PMF and 3% of patients with ET have *EZH2* mutations. However, no mutation has been reported for PV [107]. The mutation of *EZH2* has not been associated with driver mutations such as *JAK2*, *MPL*, *CALR* [108].

Spliceosome Complex Components (*SRSF2, U2AF1, SF3B1*)

SRSF2 (Serine/Arginine-Rich Splicing Factor 2)

SRSF2 (Serine/Arginine-rich Splicing Factor 2) is a protein that is encoded by *SRSF2* gene (OMIM, *600813) located on chromosome 17q25.1. The protein is a member of serine-arginine (SR) rich family of pre-mRNA splicing factors composed of 11 members that functions in pre-mRNA splicing. It has a carboxyl-terminal SR-rich domain at carboxyl terminus and a ribonucleoprotein (RNP) type RNA binding domain at amino terminus which is used to bind to the spliceosome complex [109].

SRSF2 can bind to exonic splicing enhancer on pre-mRNA and increase exon recognition, which also triggers binding of U2AF and U1 snRNP for splicing mechanism. The mutations of *SRSF2* (P95H, P95L, and P95R) are gain-of-function mutations and have been associated with MDS. It has been suggested that MDS pathogenesis is mostly caused by abnormal pre-mRNA splicing [110]. This mis-splicing may change the final product level in the cell, thus cause impaired epigenetic regulation [109]. Ernst et al. have demonstrated that 12% of the patients with MDS/MPN, and 13-17% of patients with PMF had mono- or biallelic *EZH2* mutations [8, 12]. Yoshida et al. have shown that *SRSF2* mutation (25.6%) was second only to *SF3B1* (36%), and was more common than *U2AF35* (16.9%) and *ZRSR2* (10.5%) mutations in patients with myeloid neoplasms such as MDS, t-AML, AML-MRC, and CMML [110]. Other studies have reported *SRSF2* mutations within a range of 20-53% for CMML, 0-40% in juvenile myelomonocytic leukemia (JMML), up to 40% for aCML, and between 2-9% for MDS/MPN [111].

SF3B1 (Splicing Factor 3b, Subunit 1)

SF3B1 Splicing Factor 3b, Subunit 1 is another member of polycomb group proteins and a part of spliceosome complex. This protein is encoded by *SF3B1* gene (OMIM, *605590), located on chromosome 2q33.1, and is responsible for binding of U2 snRNP to the branch point on pre-mRNA for correct splicing. In case of a mutation, this heptameric protein complex cannot recruit the spliceosome complex, which will result in formation of a truncated protein. The protein has N-terminal domain (NTD) and a carboxyl-terminal Huntingtin, elongation factor 3, protein phosphatase 2A and yeast PI3-kinase TOR1 (HEAT) repeat domain (HD) [112].

Mutations of *SF3BP1* has been shown in a group of disorders including MDS, and MPNs including CLL and PMF [112, 113]. The mutations are usually heterozygous missense mutations and more than half of them constitute K700E (c.2098A>G) mutation in patients with CLL with ring sideroblasts. In addition, other mutations such as E622D, Y623C, R625H (also R625G, C or L), N626D, H662Q or D, K666E (also K666N, R or T) and I704V (also I704N) can be detected in patients with MDS-RS [112]. Nevertheless, mutations of *SF3B1* (mentioned above) have also been emphasized in patients with PMF, which leads to the conclusion that impaired pre-mRNA splicing has a major role in development of myeloid disorders.

Transcriptional Regulators (*RUNX1*)

RUNX1 (Runt-Related Transcription Factor 1)

RUNX1 (Runt-Related Transcription Factor 1, also known as Core Binding Factor (CBF), and Acute Myeloid Leukemia 1 Protein (AML1)), is a transcription factor. It has a heterodimeric structure and binds with the core elements of promoters and enhancers through the core consensus binding domain, which is mostly 5'-TGTGGT-3', or rarely 5'-TGCGGT-3'.

The protein has two domains, which are the runt homology domain (RHD) and the transactivation domain (TAD). These domains are functional in DNA binding and interacting with other proteins. While it binds DNA as a monomer, it increases the binding efficacy if it is bound through core binding factor β (CBFβ).

The protein is encoded by *RUNX1* gene (OMIM, *151385) that is located on chromosome 21q22.12, and is the subunit of CBF. The function of this protein is to take role in hematopoiesis and differentiation of hematopoietic stem cells to lymphoid and myeloid cell lines. In addition, it plays role in TGFβ and p53 pathways, cell cycle regulation, and ribosome biogenesis [114]. The mutated gene has been shown to disrupt the differentiation process. Mutations of *RUNX1* have been rarely reported in PV (2%), ET (2%) and PMF (3%) [86]. On the other hand, a number of mutations have been associated with other hematological malignancies, such as MDS, AML, ALL, CML [114]. Nevertheless, inv(21)(q21;q22) has been reported in CMML. Mutations of *RUNX1* are generally accompanied by other mutations, such as *TET2, ASXL1, RB1, IDH1, WT1, SRSF2*, etc. [115].

CONCLUSION

Myeloproliferative neoplasms are a group of complex disorders which are affected by genetic, epigenetic and environmental changes. Mutations and larger chromosomal aberrations may change the severity of the disorder, as well as the life quality of the patient and health care takers. Since advancements of technology are used in every aspect of life, including health, newly developed techniques such as next-generation sequencing (NGS) will help the researchers and the health professionals to diagnose and treat the diseases in earlier stages. In the future, genetic tests along with more conventional methods will be used ever-increasingly for further diagnosis of these complex disorders.

REFERENCES

[1] Dean, L. *Blood groups and red cell antigens* In: Dean L, editor. 1. Bethesda, MD.: National Center for Biotechnology Information (US), 2005.

[2] Arber, DA; Orazi, A; Hasserjian, R; Thiele, J; Borowitz, MJ; Le Beau, MM; et al. The 2016 revision to the World Health Organization classification of myeloid neoplasms and acute leukemia. *Blood.*, 2016, 127(20), 2391-405.

[3] Bellanne-Chantelot, C; Moraes, GR; Schmaltz-Panneau, B; Marty, C; Vainchenker, W; Plo, I. Germline genetic factors in the pathogenesis of myeloproliferative neoplasms. *Blood Reviews.*, 2020, 42.

[4] Palomo, L; Meggendorfer, M; Hutter, S; Twardziok, S; Adema, V; Fuhrmann, I; et al. Molecular landscape and clonal architecture of adult myelodysplastic/myeloproliferative neoplasms. *Blood.*, 2020, 136(16), 1851-62.

[5] Barbui, T; Thiele, J; Gisslinger, H; Finazzi, G; Vannucchi, AM; Tefferi, A. The 2016 revision of WHO classification of myeloproliferative neoplasms: Clinical and molecular advances. *Blood Rev.*, 2016, 30(6), 453-9.

[6] Gilani, JA; Ashfaq, MA; Mansoor, AE; Abdul Jabbar, A; Siddiqui, T; Khan, M. Overview of the Mutational Landscape in Primary Myelofibrosis and Advances in Novel Therapeutics. *Asian Pac J Cancer Prev.*, 2019, 20(6), 1691-9.

[7] Barbui, T; Thiele, J; Gisslinger, H; Kvasnicka, HM; Vannucchi, AM; Guglielmelli, P; et al. The 2016 WHO classification and diagnostic criteria for myeloproliferative neoplasms: document summary and in-depth discussion. *Blood Cancer Journal.*, 2018, 8.

[8] Tefferi, A. Primary myelofibrosis: 2021 update on diagnosis, risk-stratification and management. *American Journal of Hematology.*, 2021, 96(1), 145-62.

[9] Takenaka, K; Shimoda, K; Akashi, K. Recent advances in the diagnosis and management of primary myelofibrosis. *Korean Journal of Internal Medicine.*, 2018, 33(4), 679-90.

[10] Skov, V; Riley, CH; Thomassen, M; Larsen, TS; Jensen, MK; Bjerrum, OW; et al. Whole blood transcriptional profiling reveals significant down-regulation of human leukocyte antigen class I and II genes in essential thrombocythemia, polycythemia vera and myelofibrosis. *Leukemia & Lymphoma.*, 2013, 54(10), 2269-73.

[11] Skoda, RC; Duek, A; Grisouard, J. Pathogenesis of myeloproliferative neoplasms. *Exp Hematol.*, 2015, 43(8), 599-608.

[12] Ernst, T; Chase, AJ; Score, J; Hidalgo-Curtis, CE; Bryant, C; Jones, AV; et al. Inactivating mutations of the histone methyltransferase gene EZH2 in myeloid disorders. *Nat Genet.*, 2010, 42(8), 722-6.

[13] Reilly, JT. Pathogenetic insight and prognostic information from standard and molecular cytogenetic studies in the BCR-ABL-negative myeloproliferative neoplasms (MPNs). *Leukemia.*, 2008, 22(10), 1818-27.

[14] Tefferi, A; Nicolosi, M; Mudireddy, M; Lasho, TL; Gangat, N; Begna, KH; et al. Revised cytogenetic risk stratification in primary myelofibrosis: analysis based on 1002 informative patients. *Leukemia.*, 2018, 32(5), 1189-99.

[15] Cervantes, F; Dupriez, B; Pereira, A; Passamonti, F; Reilly, JT; Morra, E; et al. New prognostic scoring system for primary myelofibrosis based on a study of the International Working Group for Myelofibrosis Research and Treatment. *Blood.*, 2009, 113(13), 2895-901.

[16] Passamonti, F; Cervantes, F; Vannucchi, AM; Morra, E; Rumi, E; Pereira, A; et al. A dynamic prognostic model to predict survival in primary myelofibrosis: a study by the IWG-MRT (International Working Group for Myeloproliferative Neoplasms Research and Treatment). *Blood.*, 2010, 115(9), 1703-8.

[17] Lu, X; Chang, R. *Polycythemia Vera*. StatPearls. Treasure Island (FL): StatPearls Publishing Copyright © 2021, StatPearls Publishing LLC., 2021.

[18] Panani, AD. Cytogenetic and molecular aspects of Philadelphia negative chronic myeloproliferative disorders: clinical implications. *Cancer Lett.*, 2007, 255(1), 12-25.

[19] Tang, G; Hidalgo Lopez, JE; Wang, SA; Hu, S; Ma, J; Pierce, S; et al. Characteristics and clinical significance of cytogenetic abnormalities in polycythemia vera. *Haematologica.*, 2017, 102(9), 1511-8.

[20] Kim, SY; Koo, M; Park, Y; Kim, H; Choi, Q; Song, IC; et al. Cytogenetic evolution in myeloproliferative neoplasms with different molecular abnormalities. *Blood Cells Mol Dis.*, 2019, 77, 120-8.

[21] Chuzi, S; Stein, BL. Essential thrombocythemia: a review of the clinical features, diagnostic challenges, and treatment modalities in the era of molecular discovery. *Leuk Lymphoma.*, 2017, 58(12), 2786-98.

[22] Tefferi, A; Barbui, T. Polycythemia vera and essential thrombocythemia: 2021 update on diagnosis, risk-stratification and management. *Am J Hematol.*, 2020, 95(12), 1599-613.
[23] Barbui, T; Thiele, J; Ferrari, A; Vannucchi, AM; Tefferi, A. The new WHO classification for essential thrombocythemia calls for revision of available evidences. *Blood Cancer J.*, 2020, 10(2), 22.
[24] Lin, Q; Mao, L; Shao, L; Zhu, L; Han, Q; Zhu, H; et al. Global; Regional, and National Burden of Chronic Myeloid Leukemia, 1990-2017: A Systematic Analysis for the Global Burden of Disease Study 2017. *Front Oncol.*, 2020, 10, 580759.
[25] Kuru, D; Tarkan Argüden, Y; Ar, MC; Çırakoğlu, A; Öngören, Ş; Yılmaz, Ş; et al. Variant Philadelphia translocations with different breakpoints in six chronic myeloid leukemia patients. *Turk J Haematol.*, 2011, 28(3), 186-92.
[26] Weerkamp, F; Dekking, E; Ng, YY; van der Velden, VH; Wai, H; Böttcher, S; et al. Flow cytometric immunobead assay for the detection of BCR-ABL fusion proteins in leukemia patients. *Leukemia.*, 2009, 23(6), 1106-17.
[27] Li, S; Ilaria, RL; Jr. Million, RP; Daley, GQ; Van Etten, RA. The P190, P210, and P230 forms of the BCR/ABL oncogene induce a similar chronic myeloid leukemia-like syndrome in mice but have different lymphoid leukemogenic activity. *J Exp Med.*, 1999, 189(9), 1399-412.
[28] Kang, ZJ; Liu, YF; Xu, LZ; Long, ZJ; Huang, D; Yang, Y; et al. The Philadelphia chromosome in leukemogenesis. *Chin J Cancer.*, 2016, 35, 48.
[29] Braun, TP; Eide, CA; Druker, BJ. Response and Resistance to BCR-ABL1-Targeted Therapies. *Cancer Cell.*, 2020, 37(4), 530-42.
[30] Jabbour, E; Kantarjian, H. Chronic myeloid leukemia: 2018 update on diagnosis, therapy and monitoring. *Am J Hematol.*, 2018, 93(3), 442-59.
[31] Bonifacio, M; Stagno, F; Scaffidi, L; Krampera, M; Di Raimondo, F. Management of Chronic Myeloid Leukemia in Advanced Phase. *Front Oncol.*, 2019, 9, 1132.
[32] Kanegae, MP; Ximenes, VF; Falcão, RP; Colturato, VA; de Mattos, ER; Brunetti, IL; et al. Chemiluminescent determination of

leukocyte alkaline phosphatase: an advantageous alternative to the cytochemical assay. *J Clin Lab Anal.*, 2007, 21(2), 91-6.

[33] Baccarani, M; Deininger, MW; Rosti, G; Hochhaus, A; Soverini, S; Apperley, JF; et al. European Leukemia Net recommendations for the management of chronic myeloid leukemia: 2013. *Blood.*, 2013, 122(6), 872-84.

[34] O'Hare, T; Shakespeare, WC; Zhu, X; Eide, CA; Rivera, VM; Wang, F; et al. AP24534, a pan-BCR-ABL inhibitor for chronic myeloid leukemia, potently inhibits the T315I mutant and overcomes mutation-based resistance. *Cancer Cell.*, 2009, 16(5), 401-12.

[35] Burchert, A; Wang, Y; Cai, D; von Bubnoff, N; Paschka, P; Muller-Brusselbach, S; et al. Compensatory PI3-kinase/Akt/mTor activation regulates imatinib resistance development. *Leukemia.*, 2005, 19(10), 1774-82.

[36] Warsch, W; Kollmann, K; Eckelhart, E; Fajmann, S; Cerny-Reiterer, S; Holbl, A; et al. High STAT5 levels mediate imatinib resistance and indicate disease progression in chronic myeloid leukemia. *Blood.*, 2011, 117(12), 3409-20.

[37] Pardanani, AD; Levine, RL; Lasho, T; Pikman, Y; Mesa, RA; Wadleigh, M; et al. MPL515 mutations in myeloproliferative and other myeloid disorders: a study of 1182 patients. *Blood.*, 2006, 108(10), 3472-6.

[38] Tefferi, A; Patnaik, MM; Pardanani, A. Eosinophilia: secondary, clonal and idiopathic. *Br J Haematol.*, 2006, 133(5), 468-92.

[39] Helbig, G; Soja, A; Bartkowska-Chrobok, A; Kyrcz-Krzemien, S. Chronic eosinophilic leukemia-not otherwise specified has a poor prognosis with unresponsiveness to conventional treatment and high risk of acute transformation. *Am J Hematol.*, 2012, 87(6), 643-5.

[40] Ogbogu, PU; Rosing, DR; Horne, MK. 3rd. Cardiovascular manifestations of hypereosinophilic syndromes. *Immunol Allergy Clin North Am.*, 2007, 27(3), 457-75.

[41] Tefferi, A; Gotlib, J; Pardanani, A. Hypereosinophilic syndrome and clonal eosinophilia: point-of-care diagnostic algorithm and treatment update. *Mayo Clin Proc.*, 2010, 85(2), 158-64.

[42] Gotlib, J. World Health Organization-defined eosinophilic disorders: 2017 update on diagnosis, risk stratification, and management. *Am J Hematol.*, 2017, 92(11), 1243-59.
[43] Klion, AD; Robyn, J; Maric, I; Fu, W; Schmid, L; Lemery, S; et al. Relapse following discontinuation of imatinib mesylate therapy for FIP1L1/PDGFRA-positive chronic eosinophilic leukemia: implications for optimal dosing. *Blood.*, 2007, 110(10), 3552-6.
[44] Lierman, E; Michaux, L; Beullens, E; Pierre, P; Marynen, P; Cools, J; et al. FIP1L1-PDGFRalpha D842V, a novel panresistant mutant, emerging after treatment of FIP1L1-PDGFRalpha T674I eosinophilic leukemia with single agent sorafenib. *Leukemia.*, 2009, 23(5), 845-51.
[45] Korkmaz, S. Non-classic myeloproliferative neoplasms: Are e really aware of these rare diseases in daily practice?. *EMJ.*, 2017, 2(3).
[46] Rollison, DE; Howlader, N; Smith, MT; Strom, SS; Merritt, WD; Ries, LA; et al. Epidemiology of myelodysplastic syndromes and chronic myeloproliferative disorders in the United States, 2001-2004, using data from the NAACCR and SEER programs. *Blood.*, 2008, 112(1), 45-52.
[47] Swerdlow, SH; Campo, E; Pileri, SA; Harris, NL; Stein, H; Siebert, R; et al. The 2016 revision of the World Health Organization classification of lymphoid neoplasms. *Blood.*, 2016, 127(20), 2375-90.
[48] Gianelli, U; Cattaneo, D; Bossi, A; Cortinovis, I; Boiocchi L; Liu YC; et al. The myeloproliferative neoplasms, unclassifiable: clinical and pathological considerations. *Mod Pathol.*, 2017, 30(2), 169-79.
[49] Kim, SY; Im, K; Park, SN; Kwon, J; Kim, JA; Lee, DS. CALR, JAK2, and MPL mutation profiles in patients with four different subtypes of myeloproliferative neoplasms: primary myelofibrosis, essential thrombocythemia, polycythemia vera, and myeloproliferative neoplasm, unclassifiable. *Am J Clin Pathol.*, 2015, 143(5), 635-44.
[50] Bose, P; Nazha, A; Komrokji, RS; Patel, KP; Pierce, SA; Al-Ali, N; et al. Mutational landscape of myelodysplastic/myeloproliferative neoplasm-unclassifiable. *Blood.,* 2018, 132(19), 2100-3.

[51] Elena, C; Galli, A; Such, E; Meggendorfer, M; Germing, U; Rizzo, E; et al. Integrating clinical features and genetic lesions in the risk assessment of patients with chronic myelomonocytic leukemia. *Blood.*, 2016, 128(10), 1408-17.

[52] Patnaik, MM; Barraco, D; Lasho, TL; Finke, CM; Reichard, K; Hoversten, KP; et al. Targeted next generation sequencing and identification of risk factors in World Health Organization defined atypical chronic myeloid leukemia. *Am J Hematol.*, 2017, 92(6), 542-8.

[53] Piazza, R; Valletta, S; Winkelmann, N; Redaelli, S; Spinelli, R; Pirola, A; et al. Recurrent SETBP1 mutations in atypical chronic myeloid leukemia. *Nat Genet.*, 2013, 45(1), 18-24.

[54] Broseus, J; Alpermann, T; Wulfert, M; Florensa Brichs, L; Jeromin, S; Lippert, E; et al. Age, JAK2(V617F) and SF3B1 mutations are the main predicting factors for survival in refractory anaemia with ring sideroblasts and marked thrombocytosis. *Leukemia.*, 2013, 27(9), 1826-31.

[55] Patnaik, MM; Lasho, TL; Finke, CM; Hanson, CA; King, RL; Ketterling, RP; et al. Predictors of survival in refractory anemia with ring sideroblasts and thrombocytosis (RARS-T) and the role of next-generation sequencing. *Am J Hematol.*, 2016, 91(5), 492-8.

[56] Kralovics, R; Passamonti, F; Buser, AS; Teo, SS; Tiedt, R; Passweg, JR; et al. A gain-of-function mutation of JAK2 in myeloproliferative disorders. *N Engl J Med.*, 2005, 352(17), 1779-90.

[57] Ugo, V; James, C; Vainchenker, W. [A unique clonal JAK2 mutation leading to constitutive signalling causes polycythaemia vera]. *Med Sci* (Paris)., 2005, 21(6-7), 669-70.

[58] Babon, JJ; Lucet, IS; Murphy, JM; Nicola, NA; Varghese, LN. The molecular regulation of Janus kinase (JAK) activation. *Biochem J.*, 2014, 462(1), 1-13.

[59] Lim, CP; Cao, X. Structure, function, and regulation of STAT proteins. *Mol Biosyst.*, 2006, 2(11), 536-50.

[60] Ferrao, R; Lupardus, PJ. The Janus Kinase (JAK) FERM and SH2 Domains: Bringing Specificity to JAK-Receptor Interactions. *Front Endocrinol* (Lausanne)., 2017, 8, 71.

[61] Saharinen, P; Takaluoma, K; Silvennoinen, O. Regulation of the Jak2 tyrosine kinase by its pseudokinase domain. *Mol Cell Biol.*, 2000, 20(10), 3387-95.
[62] Ungureanu, D; Wu, J; Pekkala, T; Niranjan, Y; Young, C; Jensen, ON; et al. The pseudokinase domain of JAK2 is a dual-specificity protein kinase that negatively regulates cytokine signaling. *Nat Struct Mol Biol.*, 2011, 18(9), 971-6.
[63] Scott, LM; Tong, W; Levine, RL; Scott, MA; Beer, PA; Stratton, MR; et al. JAK2 exon 12 mutations in polycythemia vera and idiopathic erythrocytosis. *N Engl J Med.*, 2007, 356(5), 459-68.
[64] Staerk, J; Defour, JP; Pecquet, C; Leroy, E; Antoine-Poirel, H; Brett, I; et al. Orientation-specific signalling by thrombopoietin receptor dimers. *Embo j.*, 2011, 30(21), 4398-413.
[65] Tefferi, A; Pardanani, A. Myeloproliferative Neoplasms: A Contemporary Review. *JAMA Oncol.*, 2015, 1(1), 97-105.
[66] Defour, JP; Itaya, M; Gryshkova, V; Brett, IC; Pecquet, C; Sato, T; et al. Tryptophan at the transmembrane-cytosolic junction modulates thrombopoietin receptor dimerization and activation. *Proc Natl Acad Sci U S A.*, 2013, 110(7), 2540-5.
[67] Pecquet, C; Staerk, J; Chaligné, R; Goss, V; Lee, KA; Zhang, X; et al. Induction of myeloproliferative disorder and myelofibrosis by thrombopoietin receptor W515 mutants is mediated by cytosolic tyrosine 112 of the receptor. *Blood.*, 2010, 115(5), 1037-48.
[68] Pikman, Y; Lee, BH; Mercher, T; McDowell, E; Ebert, BL; Gozo, M; et al. MPLW515L is a novel somatic activating mutation in myelofibrosis with myeloid metaplasia. *PLoS Med.*, 2006, 3(7), e270.
[69] Elsayed, AG; Ranavaya, A; Jamil, MO. MPL Y252H anMd PL F126fs mutations in essential thrombocythemia: Case series and review of literature. *Hematol Rep.*, 2019, 11(1), 7868.
[70] Lu, YC; Weng, WC; Lee, H. Functional roles of calreticulin in cancer biology. *Biomed Res Int.*, 2015, 2015, 526524.
[71] Gelebart, P; Opas, M; Michalak, M. Calreticulin, a Ca2+-binding chaperone of the endoplasmic reticulum. *Int J Biochem Cell Biol.*, 2005, 37(2), 260-6.

[72] Michalak, M; Groenendyk, J; Szabo, E; Gold, LI; Opas, M. Calreticulin, a multi-process calcium-buffering chaperone of the endoplasmic reticulum. *Biochem J.*, 2009, 417(3), 651-66.
[73] Varricchio, L; Falchi, M; Dall'Ora, M; De Benedittis, C; Ruggeri, A; Uversky, VN; et al. Calreticulin: Challenges Posed by the Intrinsically Disordered Nature of Calreticulin to the Study of Its Function. *Front Cell Dev Biol.*, 2017, 5, 96.
[74] Michalak, M; Corbett, EF; Mesaeli, N; Nakamura, K; Opas, M. Calreticulin: one protein, one gene, many functions. *Biochem J.*, 1999, 344 Pt 2(Pt 2), 281-92.
[75] Klampfl, T; Gisslinger, H; Harutyunyan, AS; Nivarthi, H; Rumi, E; Milosevic, JD; et al. Somatic mutations of calreticulin in myeloproliferative neoplasms. *N Engl J Med.*, 2013, 369(25), 2379-90.
[76] How, J; Hobbs, GS; Mullally, A. Mutant calreticulin in myeloproliferative neoplasms. *Blood.*, 2019, 134(25), 2242-8.
[77] Luo, W; Yu, Z. Calreticulin (CALR) mutation in myeloproliferative neoplasms (MPNs). *Stem Cell Investig.*, 2015, 2, 16.
[78] Nangalia, J; Massie, CE; Baxter, EJ; Nice, FL; Gundem, G; Wedge, DC; et al. Somatic CALR mutations in myeloproliferative neoplasms with nonmutated JAK2. *N Engl J Med.*, 2013, 369(25), 2391-405.
[79] Beekman, R; Touw, IP. G-CSF and its receptor in myeloid malignancy. *Blood.*, 2010, 115(25), 5131-6.
[80] Dong, F; van Buitenen, C; Pouwels, K; Hoefsloot, LH; Löwenberg, B; Touw, IP. Distinct cytoplasmic regions of the human granulocyte colony-stimulating factor receptor involved in induction of proliferation and maturation. *Mol Cell Biol.*, 1993, 13(12), 7774-81.
[81] Metcalf, D. The granulocyte-macrophage colony-stimulating factors. *Science.*, 1985, 229(4708), 16-22.
[82] Touw, IP; van de Geijn, GJ. Granulocyte colony-stimulating factor and its receptor in normal myeloid cell development, leukemia and related blood cell disorders. *Front Biosci.*, 2007, 12, 800-15.
[83] Price, A; Druhan, LJ; Lance, A; Clark, G; Vestal, CG; Zhang, Q; et al. T618I CSF3R mutations in chronic neutrophilic leukemia induce oncogenic signals through aberrant trafficking and

constitutive phosphorylation of the O-glycosylated receptor form. *Biochem Biophys Res Commun.*, 2020, 523(1), 208-13.

[84] Guglielmelli, P; Lasho, TL; Rotunno, G; Score, J; Mannarelli, C; Pancrazzi, A; et al. The number of prognostically detrimental mutations and prognosis in primary myelofibrosis: an international study of 797 patients. *Leukemia.*, 2014, 28(9), 1804-10.

[85] Lundberg, P; Karow, A; Nienhold, R; Looser, R; Hao-Shen, H; Nissen, I; et al. Clonal evolution and clinical correlates of somatic mutations in myeloproliferative neoplasms. *Blood.*, 2014, 123(14), 2220-8.

[86] Grabek, J; Straube, J; Bywater, M; Lane, SW. MPN: The Molecular Drivers of Disease Initiation, Progression and Transformation and their Effect on Treatment. *Cells.*, 2020, 9(8).

[87] Yang, L; Rau, R; Goodell, MA. DNMT3A in haematological malignancies. *Nat Rev Cancer.*, 2015, 15(3), 152-65.

[88] Ley, TJ; Ding, L; Walter, MJ; McLellan, MD; Lamprecht, T; Larson, DE; et al. DNMT3A mutations in acute myeloid leukemia. *N Engl J Med.*, 2010, 363(25), 2424-33.

[89] Solary, E; Bernard, OA; Tefferi, A; Fuks, F; Vainchenker, W. The Ten-Eleven Translocation-2 (TET2) gene in hematopoiesis and hematopoietic diseases. *Leukemia.*, 2014, 28(3), 485-96.

[90] Cimmino, L; Dolgalev, I; Wang, Y; Yoshimi, A; Martin, GH; Wang, J; et al. Restoration of TET2 Function Blocks Aberrant Self-Renewal and Leukemia Progression. *Cell.*, 2017, 170(6), 1079-95 e20.

[91] Moran-Crusio, K; Reavie, L; Shih, A; Abdel-Wahab, O; Ndiaye-Lobry, D; Lobry, C; et al. Tet2 loss leads to increased hematopoietic stem cell self-renewal and myeloid transformation. *Cancer Cell.*, 2011, 20(1), 11-24.

[92] Feng, Y; Li, X; Cassady, K; Zou, Z; Zhang, X. TET2 Function in Hematopoietic Malignancies, Immune Regulation, and DNA Repair. *Front Oncol.*, 2019, 9, 210.

[93] Jan, M; Snyder, TM; Corces-Zimmerman, MR; Vyas, P; Weissman, IL; Quake, SR; et al. Clonal evolution of preleukemic hematopoietic stem cells precedes human acute myeloid leukemia. *Sci Transl Med.*, 2012, 4(149), 149ra18.

[94] Beer, PA; Delhommeau, F; LeCouedic, JP; Dawson, MA; Chen, E; Bareford, D; et al. Two routes to leukemic transformation after a JAK2 mutation-positive myeloproliferative neoplasm. *Blood.*, 2010, 115(14), 2891-900.

[95] Gelsi-Boyer, V; Brecqueville, M; Devillier, R; Murati, A; Mozziconacci, MJ; Birnbaum, D. Mutations in ASXL1 are associated with poor prognosis across the spectrum of malignant myeloid diseases. *J Hematol Oncol.*, 2012, 5, 12.

[96] Shen, Q; Zhang, Q; Shi, Y; Shi, Q; Jiang, Y; Gu, Y; et al. Tet2 promotes pathogen infection-induced myelopoiesis through mRNA oxidation. *Nature.*, 2018, 554(7690), 123-7.

[97] Xu, X; Zhao, J; Xu, Z; Peng, B; Huang, Q; Arnold, E; et al. Structures of human cytosolic NADP-dependent isocitrate dehydrogenase reveal a novel self-regulatory mechanism of activity. *J Biol Chem.*, 2004, 279(32), 33946-57.

[98] Molenaar, RJ; Maciejewski, JP; Wilmink, JW; van Noorden, CJF. Wild-type and mutated IDH1/2 enzymes and therapy responses. *Oncogene.*, 2018, 37(15), 1949-60.

[99] Lu, C; Ward, PS; Kapoor, GS; Rohle, D; Turcan, S; Abdel-Wahab, O; et al. IDH mutation impairs histone demethylation and results in a block to cell differentiation. *Nature.*, 2012, 483(7390), 474-8.

[100] Asada, S; Fujino, T; Goyama, S; Kitamura, T. The role of ASXL1 in hematopoiesis and myeloid malignancies. *Cell Mol Life Sci.*, 2019, 76(13), 2511-23.

[101] Yang, H; Kurtenbach, S; Guo, Y; Lohse, I; Durante, MA; Li, J; et al. Gain of function of ASXL1 truncating protein in the pathogenesis of myeloid malignancies. *Blood.*, 2018, 131(3), 328-41.

[102] Abdel-Wahab, O; Adli, M; LaFave, LM; Gao, J; Hricik, T; Shih, AH; et al. ASXL1 mutations promote myeloid transformation through loss of PRC2-mediated gene repression. *Cancer Cell.*, 2012, 22(2), 180-93.

[103] Balasubramani, A; Larjo, A; Bassein, JA; Chang, X; Hastie, RB; Togher, SM; et al. Cancer-associated ASXL1 mutations may act as gain-of-function mutations of the ASXL1-BAP1 complex. *Nat Commun.*, 2015, 6, 7307.

[104] Gan, L; Yang, Y; Li, Q; Feng, Y; Liu, T; Guo, W. Epigenetic regulation of cancer progression by EZH2: from biological insights to therapeutic potential. *Biomark Res.*, 2018, 6, 10.

[105] Cao, Q; Yu, J; Dhanasekaran, SM; Kim, JH; Mani, RS; Tomlins, SA; et al. Repression of E-cadherin by the polycomb group protein EZH2 in cancer. *Oncogene.*, 2008, 27(58), 7274-84.

[106] Ma, DN; Chai, ZT; Zhu, XD; Zhang, N; Zhan, DH; Ye, BG; et al. MicroRNA-26a suppresses epithelial-mesenchymal transition in human hepatocellular carcinoma by repressing enhancer of zeste homolog 2. *J Hematol Oncol.*, 2016, 9, 1.

[107] Tefferi, A; Lasho, TL; Guglielmelli, P; Finke, CM; Rotunno, G; Elala, Y; et al. Targeted deep sequencing in polycythemia vera and essential thrombocythemia. *Blood Adv.*, 2016, 1(1), 21-30.

[108] Lasho, TL; Mudireddy, M; Finke, CM; Hanson, CA; Ketterling, RP; Szuber, N; et al. Targeted next-generation sequencing in blast phase myeloproliferative neoplasms. *Blood Adv.*, 2018, 2(4), 370-80.

[109] Masaki, S; Ikeda, S; Hata, A; Shiozawa, Y; Kon, A; Ogawa, S; et al. Myelodysplastic Syndrome-Associated SRSF2 Mutations Cause Splicing Changes by Altering Binding Motif Sequences. *Front Genet.*, 2019, 10, 338.

[110] Yoshida, K; Sanada, M; Shiraishi, Y; Nowak, D; Nagata, Y; Yamamoto, R; et al. Frequent pathway mutations of splicing machinery in myelodysplasia. *Nature.*, 2011, 478(7367), 64-9.

[111] Aujla, A; Linder, K; Iragavarapu, C; Karass, M; Liu, D. SRSF2 mutations in myelodysplasia/myeloproliferative neoplasms. *Biomark Res.*, 2018, 6, 29.

[112] Foy, A; McMullin, MF. Somatic SF3B1 mutations in myelodysplastic syndrome with ring sideroblasts and chronic lymphocytic leukaemia. *J Clin Pathol.*, 2019, 72(11), 778-82.

[113] Lasho, TL; Finke, CM; Hanson, CA; Jimma, T; Knudson, RA; Ketterling, RP; et al. SF3B1 mutations in primary myelofibrosis: clinical; histopathology and genetic correlates among 155 patients. *Leukemia,.* 2012, 26(5), 1135-7.

[114] Sood, R; Kamikubo, Y; Liu, P. Role of RUNX1 in hematological malignancies. *Blood.*, 2017, 129(15), 2070-82.
[115] Yokota, A; Huo, L; Lan, F; Wu, J; Huang, G. The Clinical, Molecular, and Mechanistic Basis of RUNX1 Mutations Identified in Hematological Malignancies. *Mol Cells.*, 2020, 43(2), 145-52.

In: New Research on Hematological ...
Editor: David K. Gioia

ISBN: 978-1-53619-955-0
© 2021 Nova Science Publishers, Inc.

Chapter 2

TREATMENT OF MYELOID HEMATOLOGIC MALIGNANCIES WITH ISOCITRATE DEHYDROGENASE MUTATIONS BY INHIBITORS OF THIS ENZYME

Ota Fuchs[*]
Institute of Hematology and Blood Transfusion,
Prague, Czech Republic

ABSTRACT

Isocitrate dehydrogenase (IDH) is an important metabolic enzyme in the Krebs Cycle that catalyzes the conversion of isocitrate to α-ketoglutarate. The mutant IDH protein leads to an accumulation of 2-hydroxyglutarate, a metabolite with oncogenic activity via epigenetic mechanisms. This metabolite is similar to α-ketoglutarate and competitively inhibits α-ketoglutarate-dependent enzymes, alters DNA and histone methylation, and impairs cellular growth and differentiation. Recurrent IDH1 and IDH2 mutations occur in about 20% of patients with acute myeloid leukemia (AML) and 5% of patients with myelodysplastic syndromes (MDS). Small molecule inhibitors of mutant IDH1 and IDH2 were developed and

---

[*] Corresponding Author's E-mail: Ota.Fuchs@uhkt.cz.

used in pre-clinical and clinical studies. Two of these inhibitors, ivosidenib (AG-120, Tibsovo) and enasidenib (AG-221, Idhifa) were approved by the US Food and Drug Administration (FDA) for the treatment of newly diagnosed and relapsed/refractory IDH1 and IDH2 mutant AML, respectively. Despite the high efficacy and activity of these IDH1 and IDH2 inhibitors, monotherapy showed response rates of less than 50%. Resistance was described in some cases with co-occurring mutations in receptor tyrosine kinase FLT3, transcription factors (RUNX1, GATA-2, CEBPA), or IDH1 second-site mutation. Therefore, various therapies that use a combination of the IDH1 and IDH2 inhibitors with hypomethylating agent azacitidine were studied with better results than when monotherapy was used.

Keywords: acute myeloid leukemia, myelodysplastic syndrome, IDH1 and IDH2 mutations, 2-hydroxyglutarate, ivosidenib, enasidenib

INTRODUCTION

Genes encoding two isoforms of isocitrate dehydrogenase (*IDH1* and *IDH2*) belong to the most commonly mutated genes in AML. Recurring IDH1 and IDH2 mutations were reported in glioblastoma [1-3], and then in AML, cholangiocarcinoma, chondrosarcoma, chondromas, fibrosarcoma, astrocytoma, melanoma, and thyroid carcinoma [4-10]. Eukaryotic cells express three different forms of IDH [11]. These different isoforms of IDH are encoded by five genes in the human genome. IDH1 and IDH2 are each coded by one gene. A third isoform IDH3 is encoded by three different genes (*IDH3A*, *IDH3B*, *IDH3G*). These three genes are not significantly mutated in human cancers. Their mutations are not likely to be drivers, and therefore *IDH3* mutations will not be discussed in this chapter. The vast majority of cancer-associated mutations in *IDH1* and *IDH2* map to arginine residues within the catalytic pocket in the enzyme active sites. Mutations in *IDH1* mostly occur at arginine 132. A single amino acid substitution in this location is first of all to histidine (R132H), but also to cysteine (R132C), serine (R132S), glycine (R132G), leucine (R132L), and isoleucine (R132I). Mutations in *IDH2* occur at arginine 172 or arginine 140 predominantly as R140Q or R172K [12, 13]. Somatic mutations in either of these two genes pass on a neomorphic enzymatic activity resulting in the ability to convert α-ketoglutarate (αKG) into the oncometabolite R(-) enantiomer of the metabolite 2-hydroxyglutarate (R-2-HG) which accumulates in *IDH-* mutant human gliomas or leukemias [14-17]. Elevated concentrations of R-2-HG inhibit αKG-dependent dioxygenases, alter DNA and histone methylation, and inhibit a normal differentiation process in a manner that promotes leukemogenesis and tumorigenesis. The development of novel therapies based on the small molecule oral inhibitors of the mutant IDH1 and IDH2 enzymes led to the agreement of the United States Food and Drug Administration (US FDA) with these targeted therapies to treat *IDH* mutant malignancies [18].

THE MOLECULAR STRUCTURE OF IDH ISOZYMES, THEIR LOCALIZATION, AND FUNCTION

A human *IDH1* gene is located on chromosome 2q33.3, *IDH2* on chromosome 15q26.1, *IDH3A* on chromosome 15q25.1-q25.2, *IDH3B* on chromosome 20p13, and IDH 3γ subunit is encoded by *IDH3G* on chromosome Xq28 [19, 20]. IDH1 is localized in the cytoplasm and peroxisomes. Both IDH2 and IDH3 proteins function in the mitochondria. IDH1 and IDH2 isozymes function as homodimers and have an extensive similarity. Both IDH1 subunits contain three different domains: a large domain (residues 1 to 103 and 286 to 414), a small domain (residues 104 to 136 and 186 to 285), and a clasp domain (residues 137 to 185) [21-24]. This composition is schematically outlined in Figure 1. A deep cleft formed by the large and the small domain of one subunit and a small domain of the second subunit represents the active enzyme domain. The active enzyme domain contains also the nicotinamide adenine dinucleotide phosphate (NADP)-binding site and the isocitrate-metal ion binding site. Two domains of one subunit create a shallow cleft that controls enzyme conformation. The activity of IDH1 is controlled through the regulation of substrate (isocitrate) binding to its binding site. The structure of IDH2 is the same as that of IDH1. However, IDH2 contains, in addition, a 39 amino acid mitochondrial targeting sequence at its NH_2-terminus

(Figure 1) [22, 24, 25]. IDH3 is in contrast to IDH1 and IDH2 a heterodimer composed of the αβ and αγ subunits [26].

IDH1 catalyzes the oxidative decarboxylation of isocitrate to 2-ketoglutarate (also called α-ketoglutarate) to generate NADPH from $NADP^+$ and the reverse reaction, that is reductive carboxylation of α-ketoglutarate to isocitrate that oxidizes NADPH to $NADP^+$ [22, 24, 27]. The oxidative decarboxylation of isocitrate has two steps. In the first step, isocitrate is oxidized to an unstable oxalosuccinate with concomitant reduction of $NADP^+$ to NADPH. In the second step, the oxalosuccinate loses its β-carbonyl group that leads to αKG (Figure 2). IDH2 catalyzes the same reversible reaction within mitochondria [25, 28]. IDH3 catalyzes the conversion of NAD^+ to NADH in the mitochondrion. The α-ketoglutarate produced by IDH3 is further metabolized to succinate and NADH is used by the electron transport chain to generate ATP [29]. The reactions catalyzed by IDH1 and IDH2 are reversible in contrast to the reaction catalyzed by IDH3 (Figure 2).

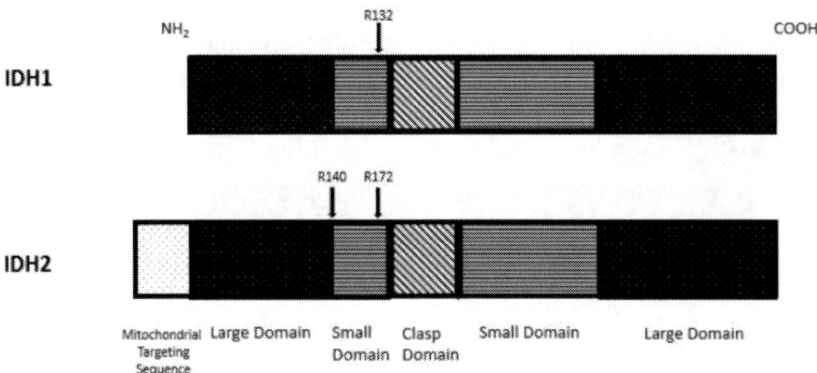

Figure 1. Structure of two isoforms of isocitrate dehydrogenase (IDH1 and IDH2). Both isoforms contain large domain, small domain and clasp domain. IDH2 contains an additional domain that contains a 39 amino acid mitochondrial targeting sequence at its NH2 terminus. The amino acid residues R132 for IDH1 and R140 with R172 for IDH2 are most frequently involved in IDH mutations. These arginine residues stabilize in unmutated IDH the substrate-binding site [22].

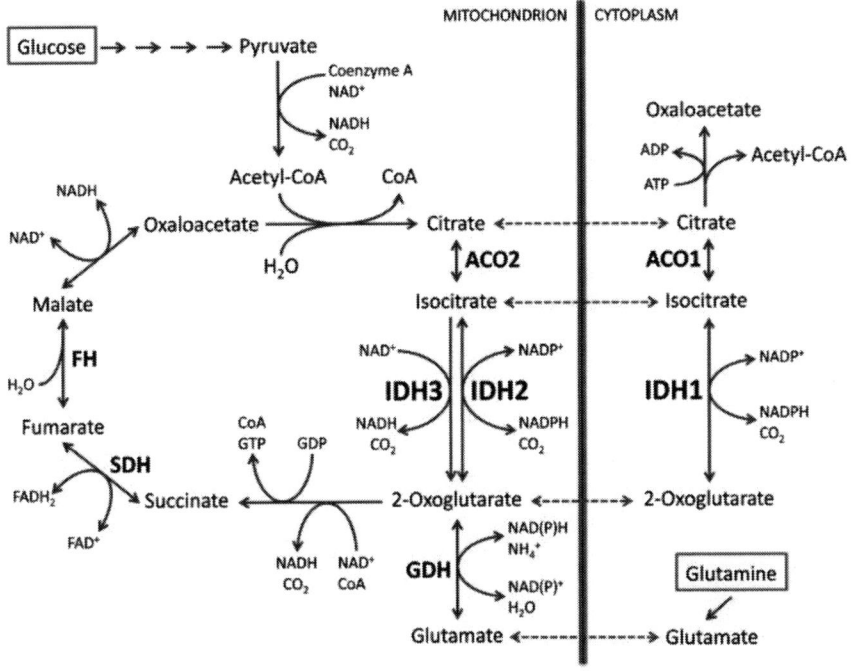

Figure 2. The participation of three different isoforms of IDH in the Krebs cycle (also known as the citric acid cycle or tricarboxylic acid cycle) that catalyzes conversion of isocitrate to α-ketoglutarate [29]. ACO-aconitase, FH-fumarate hydratase, SDH-succinate dehydrogenase, FAD-flavin adenine dinucleotide, $FADH_2$-the reduced hydroquinone form.

The Roles of 2-Hydroxyglutarate

Whole-genome sequencing performed in glioblastoma and AML with normal karyotype identified recurrent somatic mutations at Arg132 (R132) of IDH1 [1, 4]. Further studies showed that mutations in *IDH1* and *IDH2* are present in clonal myeloid disorders. The mutant IDH protein leads to accumulation of 2-hydroxyglutarate (2HG), a metabolite with oncogenic activity via epigenetic mechanisms. This metabolite is similar to α-ketoglutarate and competitively inhibits α-ketoglutarate-dependent enzymes, alters DNA and histone methylation, and impairs cellular growth and differentiation. However, hematopoietic stem cells isolated from *IDH1* R132H knock-in mice can differentiate *in vitro* and can repopulate the bone marrow of transplanted recipient mice.

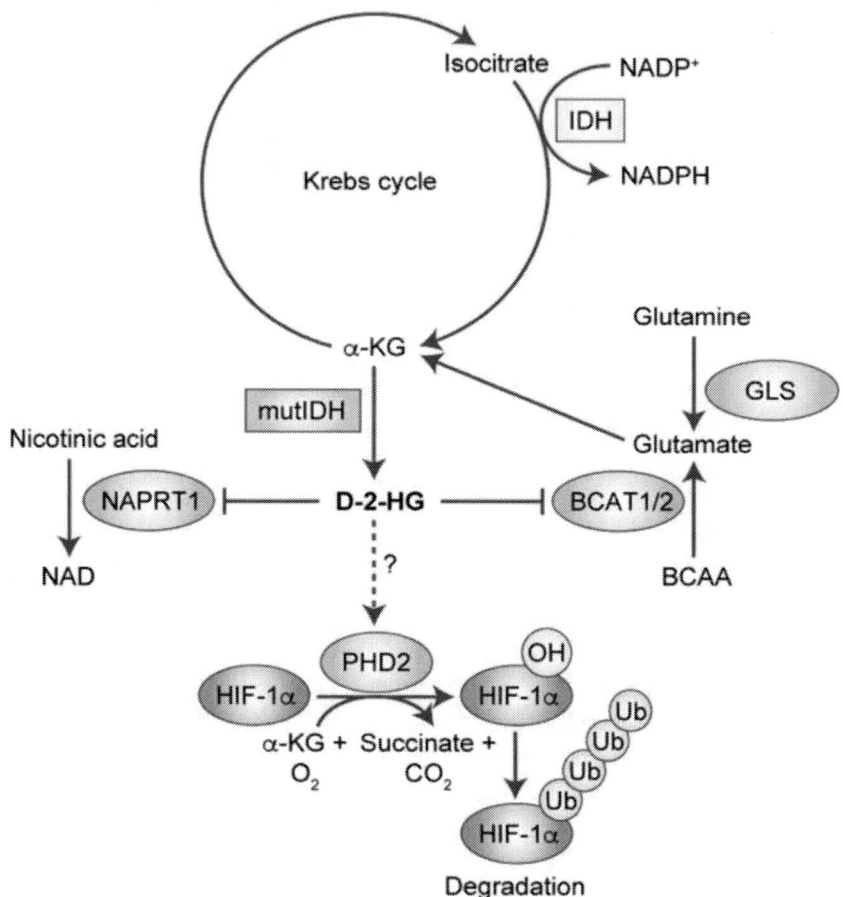

Figure 3. Metabolism changes in IDH1-mutated AML. Inhibition of Krebs cycle by exhausting α-ketoglutarate for 2-hydroxyglutarate production [3]. Metabolite such as glutamine, glutamate and branched amino acids (BCAA) serve as complementary sources to fuel cellular metabolism. BCAT-branched chain amino acid transaminase, GDH-glutamate dehydrogenase, NAPRT1-nicotinate phosphoribosyltransferase 1, PHD2-prolyl hydroxylase domain 2 enzyme.

This finding showed that other mutations cooperating with mutant IDH play an important role in the block of cellular differentiation. A five-carbon 2HG molecule contains a chiral center at the second carbon atom. Two possible enantiomers of 2HG occur: (R)-2HG/also known as (D)-2HG/and (S)-2HG/also known as (L)-2HG/ [29]. Both these chiral forms are byproducts of normal mitochondrial metabolism [29-31]. The intracellular concentration of 2HG in normal cells is very low (<0.1 mM) in contrast to *IDH* mutant cells (1-30 mM) [14, 15, 32].

The accumulation of (R)-2HG competitively inhibits multiple αKG-dependent dioxygenases [33-36]. The high concentration of 2HG in *IDH* mutant cells has been reported to activate the enzyme prolyl-hydroxylase 2 (PHD2) that inhibits hypoxia-inducible factor 1-α /HIF-1α/ (Figure 3) [35]. However, other articles suggest that PHD2 may be inhibited by increased concentration of (R)-2HG [33, 34]. Although PHD2, the enzyme hydroxylating HIF-1α is a member of αKG-dependent dioxygenases, the effect of 2HG is not clear. 2HG inhibits branched-chain amino acid transferase (BCAT1/2), consequently increasing the dependence on glutaminase to synthesize glutathione (Figure 3) [37]. Glutathione is necessary for the inhibition of reactive oxygen radicals. 2HG inhibits also nicotinate phosphoribosyltransferase 1 (NAPRT1) resulting in NAD^+ depletion (Figure 3) [38].

There are over 60 different αKG-dependent dioxygenases and two groups of these enzymes are the major targets of αKG. The histone lysine demethylase family (KDMs) containing the jumonji domain (JmjC) and the myeloid tumor suppressor TET2 (ten-eleven translocation), a member of a TET family are the major targets of 2HG (Figure 4) [11, 33, 34, 39, 40]. Both these families play important roles in regulating gene expression through post-translational histone methylation and DNA methylation. Mice with knock-in of mutant IDH^{R132H} in their hematopoietic stem and progenitor cells (HSPCs) accumulated a high level of (R)-2HG and increased levels of trimethylated H3K4, H3K9, H3K27, and H3K36, resulting in a block of hematopoietic differentiation. However, the inhibition of the TET family of 5-methylcytosine hydroxylases by (R)-2HG resulted in a hypermethylated gene signature in HSPCs [41-43]. This signature overlaps with the signature of *IDH* and *TET2-* mutated leukemic cells and is associated with an altered expression of many genes involved in cellular differentiation. Only (R)-2HG, but not (S)-2HG, is able to transform HSPCs *in vitro* and *in vivo*. However, (S)-2HG is a potent inhibitor of the TET family of 5-methylcytosine hydroxylases [34, 40].

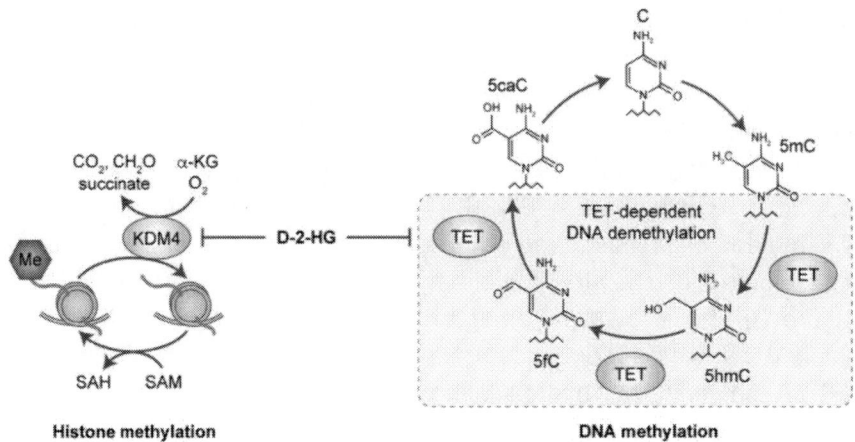

Figure 4. Mutated IDH1 affects epigenome. 2-hydroxyglutarate produced by IDH1-mutant serves as a competitive inhibitor for KDM4 or TET and therefore blocks the demethylation process in histone and nucleotide, respectively [3].

(R)-2HG also inhibits cytochrome c oxidase (COX) in the electron transport chain. This COX inhibition lowers the threshold for apoptosis, increasing *IDH* mutated cell dependence on BCL-2 for survival [44]. (R)-2HG also suppresses oxoglutarate dehydrogenase activity and decreases succinyl-coenzyme A (CoA) synthesis in conditional IDH1-R132Q-LSL (Lox-Stop-Lox) mice [45]. This model was described in preceding studies [46, 47]. The deficit of succinyl-CoA declines heme biosynthesis in *IDH1* – mutant hematopoietic cells. Erythroid differentiation is blocked in this way at the late erythroblast stage. The exogenous succinyl-CoA or 5-aminolevulinic acid releases erythropoiesis in *IDH1* – mutant hematopoietic cells. The decreased heme synthesis caused by the deficit of succinyl-CoA also inhibits heme oxygenase-1 expression and reduces biliverdin and bilirubin levels. Accumulation of reactive oxygen species then induces the cell death of *IDH1* – mutant hematopoietic cells [45].

(R)-2HG has been recently reported to exhibit anti-tumor activity. However, its effect on cancer metabolism remains largely elusive. (R)-

2HG abrogates fat-mass-and obesity-associated protein (FTO), N^6-methyladenosine (m^6A) and YTH N^6-methyladenosine RNA binding protein 2 (YTHDF2), and post-transcriptionally upregulates platelet phosphofructokinase (PFKP) and lactate dehydrogenase B (LDHB), and thereby suppresses aerobic glycolysis in leukemia cells but not in normal stem/progenitor CD34+ cells [48]. A similar study also showed anti-leukemic activity of (R)-2HG by targeting FTO, m^6A, MYC, CEBPA signaling. (R)-2HG inhibits FTO activity and increases global m^6A RNA modification in leukemia cells, which in turn decreases the stability of MYC and CEBPA transcripts, leading to the suppression of these signaling pathways [49]. (R)-2HG also acts as an immunometabolite and a mediator in T lymphocyte differentiation [31].

IDH MUTATIONS IN AGE-RELATED CLONAL HEMATOPOIESIS, MYELODYSPLASTIC SYNDROMES AND ACUTE MYELOID LEUKEMIA

Mutations in genes involved in epigenetic regulation (*IDH1*, *IDH2*, *DNMT3A*, *TET2*, *ASXL1*) are responsible for the majority of mutation-driven age-related clonal hematopoiesis (ARCH) [50-53]. The presence of ARCH was associated with an increased risk of developing AML. Especially, mutations in *IDH1*, *IDH2*, *TP53*, *DNMT3A*, *TET2*, and spliceosome genes increased the risk of developing AML [54, 55]. Myelodysplastic syndromes (MDS) constitute a group of age-associated heterogeneous clonal hematopoietic disorders characterized by ineffective hematopoiesis with peripheral cytopenias, dysplasia, and an increased risk of progression to AML [56-61]. A higher frequency of *IDH1* and *IDH2* mutations were detected in high-risk than in low-risk MDS [62-65]. Different isoforms of mutant *IDH1* and mutant *IDH2* are associated with various co-mutations. Mutant *IDH1* and mutant *IDH2-R140* are often associated with mutations in *NPM1*, *DNMT3A*, and *FLT3-ITD*. Mutant *IDH2-172* is associated with mutations in *DNMT3A* [62, 66]. An analysis of 1042 MDS patients showed *IDH2* mutations in 5.7% of cases (4.1% had *IDH2-R140* mutations and 0.1% had *IDH2-R172* mutations) and *IDH1-R132* mutations in 1.6% of MDS patients [65]. The dynamics of clonal evolution in MDS with *TET2* and *IDH* mutations to secondary AML (sAML) was studied. It was found that these mutations did not affect overall survival. *TET2* but not *IDH1* and *IDH2* mutations were associated with progression to sAML. Both *TET2* and *IDH* mutations contribute to MDS initiation and are maintained in the course of transformation to sAML [67]. The frequency of *IDH1* mutations increases in the progression from high-risk MDS to AML and also the frequency of *IDH2* mutations increases in the development of high-risk MDS and AML from low-risk MDS [68]. A prognostic significance of *IDH* mutations in AML is not clear. Several studies showed improved overall survival and/or complete remission rate in patients with *IDH* mutation, especially in the presence of *NPM1* mutation and in absence of *DNMT3A* mutation [69-73]. However, other studies did not find the prognostic impact of *IDH* mutations or they reported a negative prognostic impact for the mutant *IDH2-R172* isoform and *IDH*-mutated patients with normal karyotype and *NPM1* mutation in absence of *FLT3-ITD* [66, 74-79]. A more aggressive phenotype of myeloproliferative neoplasms (blastic phase) is also associated with mutations in IDH1 and IDH2 (up to 21%) in comparison with about 4% in the chronic phase [80, 81].

Several studies have evaluated whether *IDH1* and *IDH2* mutations are suitable markers for minimal residual disease [82-84]. The presence of *IDH1* and *IDH2* mutations together with *NPM1* mutations, but not *DNMT3A* mutations, was associated with leukemic disease and predicted relapse [82]. A further study reported 80 AML patients with *IDH1* and *IDH2* mutations at the time of the remission after inductive therapy. Persistent *IDH* mutations were detected in about 40% of these patients after one year of follow-up and these patients had an increased risk of relapse. On the other hand, 59% of patients without a detectable *IDH1* mutation and 24% of patients without a detectable *IDH2* mutation, respectively, were found. However, the relapse rate did not correlate with the persistence of *IDH* mutations [83]. The persistence of *IDH1* and *IDH2* mutations after allogeneic stem cell transplantation is a predictor of relapse [84].

Association between *IDH* mutation status and cardiac function, and risk of coronary artery disease, and cardiac dysfunction in AML patients were analyzed in the retrospective observational study [85]. A total of 363 patients with AML, 298 (82.1%) without *IDH* mutation (the control group), 65 (17.9%) had either an *IDH1* (26 AML patients/7.2%/) or an *IDH2* mutation (39 AML patients/10.7%/. Left ventricular ejection fraction (LVEF) was analyzed by echocardiography in the control group and the exposed group (AML patients with *IDH* mutation). Patients with *IDH* mutation in AML showed significantly reduced LVEF in the course of AML therapy and AML patients with *IDH1* mutation had a higher percentage of cardiovascular coronary disease at diagnosis. However, *IDH1* and *IDH2* mutations were without effect on relapse-free survival or crude overall survival [85].

Targeted Therapy for *IDH* Mutations

In recent years, small molecule, oral IDH inhibitors have shown good clinical response in AML patients. The phase 1-2 clinical trials led to the approval by the U.S. FDA of enasidenib and ivosidenib on 1 August 2017 and 20 July 2018 for the treatment of adult relapsed or refractory (R/R) AML patients. These inhibitors are also effective in newly diagnosed older AML patients (75 years or older) and in AML patients with comorbidities that block the use of intensive induction chemotherapy. Mutant IDH inhibitors represent a novel class of targeted cancer metabolism therapy that induces differentiation of proliferating cancer cells. Various combinations with intensive chemotherapy, hypomethylating agents, and other targeted therapies are studied.

Ongoing clinical trials of IDH1 inhibitors in AML and MDS are presented in Table 1. BAY1436032 is an oral small-molecule allosteric inhibitor of mutant IDH1. Monotherapy with this inhibitor reduced 2-HG level, inhibited proliferation of leukemia stem cells, and reversed the abnormal methylation of histone in AML patient-derived xenograft (PDX) mouse models [86]. Combination of BAY1436032 with azacitidine induced AML cell differentiation by regulating an EGR-GFI1-NF-κB pathway in two separate AML patient-derived xenograft (PDX) mouse models. The sequential combination treatment depleted leukemia stem cells (LSC) by 470-fold. The simultaneous combination treatment decreased LSC by 33,150-fold compared to control mice. This strong synergy is mediated through inhibition of MAP kinases (RAS/RAF) and retinoblastoma (Rb)/E2F signaling pathways.

Table 1. Clinical trials with IDH1 inhibitors in adult AML and MDS with mutant *IDH1*

Trial Identification	Disease	Phase	Drugs
NCT04013880	R/R AML	1/2	FT-2102 (olutasidenib) plus ASTX727 (DNMT inhibitor)
NCT02719574	AML	1/2	FT-2102 as single agent
			FT-2102 plus azacitidine or cytarabine
NCT03127735	advanced AML	1	BAY 1436032
NCT02074839	R/R AML, untreated AML	1	ivosidenib
NCT03013998 (The Beat AML Trial)	previously untreated AML	1/2	ivosidenib
NCT02677922	newly diagnosed AML	1/2	ivosidenib plus azacitidine
NCT03173248 (AGILE)	previously untreated AML	3	ivosidenib plus azacitidine versus placebo plus azacitidine
NCT02632708	newly diagnosed AML	1/2	ivosidenib or enasidenib plus standard chemotherapy
NCT03839771	newly diagnosed AML or MDS EB2	3	ivosidenib or enasidenib plus standard chemotherapy
NCT03471260	R/R AML	1/2	ivosidenib plus venetoclax with or without azacitidine

Quantitative RT-PCR analysis confirmed that the cell survival and proliferation genes *ELK1*, *ETS1*, and *CCND1* in the MAP kinase pathway and *E2F1*, *CCNA2*, and *CCNE1* in Rb/E2F signaling were additively suppressed. But then, the myeloid differentiation genes *PU.1*, *CEBPA*, and *GABPA* (GA binding protein alpha) were upregulated after the combination therapy [87, 88]. This work is highly relevant to the ongoing clinical trial NCT03127735 (Table 1) [89].

The structure-based design and optimization of quinoline lead compounds to identify FT-2102, a potent orally bioavailable, brain penetrant, and selective inhibitor of mutant IDH1 [90]. Olutasidenib (FT-2102) is a highly potent, selective small-molecule inhibitor of mutant IDH1 with the therapeutic potential to restore normal cellular differentiation in MDS or AML patients with mutant IDH1 [91, 92]. Azacitidine has shown synergistic effects with olutasidenib on releasing differentiation block in mutant IDH1 leukemia models *in vitro*. Olutasidenib phase 1/2 clinical trial as monotherapy and combined therapy with azacitidine or cytarabine for the treatment of adult R/R AML is ongoing (NCT02719574, Table 1). The phase 1 results indicated the efficiency and safety of the drug. The overall response rate was 33% and the complete remission rate was 14%. Thrombocytopenia, febrile neutropenia, anemia, and pneumonia were the main adverse reactions [91, 92].

After identification of an allosteric, induced pocket of IDH1^{R132H}, 3-pyrimidine-4-yl-oxazolidine-2-ones were studied as mutant IDH1 inhibitors for *in vivo* modulation of 2-HG production and potential brain penetration (for gliomas with mutant IDH1). IDH305 was discovered as a selective allosteric inhibitor of IDH1 mutation. Preclinical studies showed that it could reduce the 2-HG level and induce differentiation of AML cells with mutant IDH1 [93, 94]. A phase 1 study of IDH305 was specifically designed to evaluate the safety of IDH305 in cancers with IDH1^{R132} mutation, including 21 relapsed/refractory AML and 3 MDS. IDH305 was orally administered twice a day in continuous 21-day cycles. The starting dose was 75 mg with dose expansion to 900 mg. The most common adverse events were raised bilirubin and lipase (8.3% each) [93].

Ivosidenib (AG-120, Tibsovo®)

The prototype mutant IDH1 inhibitor AGI-5198 inhibited both biochemical and cellular production of 2-HG and induced epigenetic changes leading to the expression of genes associated with differentiation of mutant IDH1 cells [95]. However, the poor pharmaceutical properties of AGI-5198 prevented its use in clinical trials. A first-in-class mutant IDH1 inhibitor AG-120 (ivosidenib) was developed by optimization of AGI-5198 [96]. Ivosidenib (Figure 5) was approved by FDA in 2018 for the treatment of adult relapsed or refractory (R/R) AML patients as was described in the paragraph "Targeted Therapy for *IDH* Mutations" [97, 98]. Ivosidenib was also approved in 2019 as front-line therapy for newly diagnosed elderly patients 75 years or older or who are ineligible to receive intensive chemotherapy based on promising results of phase I-II clinical trials [99, 100].

The single-arm trial with 500mg ivosidenib daily in 174 adults with mutant IDH1 R/R AML and with a median follow-up of 8.3 months achieved 33% complete remission with a median duration of response of 8.2 months [97]. A phase 1 dose-escalation and dose-expansion study (NCT02074839, Table 1) of ivosidenib monotherapy in 179 patients with *IDH1*-mutated R/R AML showed the rate of complete remission or complete remission with partial hematologic recovery 30.4%, the rate of complete remission 21.6%, and the overall response rate 41.6% [101, 102]. Maximal inhibition of 2-HG in plasma and bone marrow was observed by day 14 in patients who received 500 mg daily. No additional inhibition was observed at higher doses (800 or 1200 mg daily). The mean plasma 2-HG level decreased to levels seen in healthy persons after multiple doses of ivosidenib (500 mg daily). Of the 179 patients, 177 (98.9%) had an adverse event. Diarrhea, leukocytosis, febrile neutropenia, nausea, fatigue, dyspnea, anemia, and peripheral edema were the most common adverse events. The IDH differentiation syndrome includes fever, cough, trouble breathing, leukocytosis, build-up of excess fluid around the heart and lungs, low blood pressure, and kidney failure. Differentiation syndrome can be life-threatening if not treated early. The IDH differentiation syndrome was managed by dose interruption and treatment with glucocorticoids, oral hydroxyurea, or both [101]. Treatment with ivosidenib can be associated with QTc interval prolongation [98]. The QT interval on the electrocardiogram (ECG) has gained clinical importance, primarily because prolongation of this interval can predispose to a potentially fatal ventricular arrhythmia. Therefore, patients on ivosidenib therapy should be monitored for increased risk of QTc interval prolongation [102].

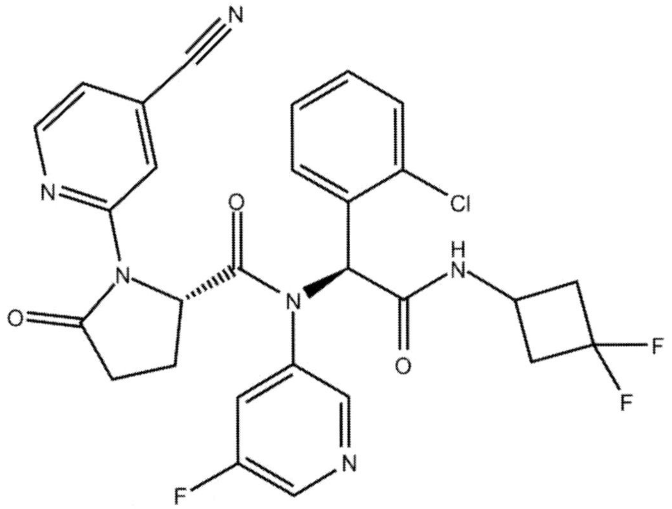

Figure 5. The chemical structure of ivosidenib. This small molecule functions as orally available inhibitor of mutated cytosolic isocitrate dehydrogenase 1 (IDH1) and was developed by Agios Pharmaceuticals and Celgene Corporation for the treatment of cancer in patients with *IDH1* mutation.

Ivosidenib monotherapy was also studied in 34 elderly (median age 76.5 years) newly diagnosed AML patients ineligible for standard therapy who received 500 mg ivosidenib daily with a median follow-up of 23.5 months[102]. Most of these patients had secondary AML (77%) and rest *de novo* AML. The overall response rate was 54.5%, complete remission 30.3%, and complete remission with partial hematologic recovery was 42.4%. Median overall survival was 12.6 months with an estimated one-year overall survival rate of 51.1%.

The most frequent co-occurring mutations at the start of ivosidenib therapy were *ASXL1*, *DNMT3A*, *RUNX1*, *SRSF2*, *TET2*, and *NRAS*.

No single mutation was significantly associated with clinical response to ivosidenib treatment. Receptor tyrosine kinase (RTK) pathway mutations (*NRAS*, *FLT3*, *PTPN11*, *KRAS*) were not observed in any of the patients achieving complete remission and complete remission with partial hematologic recovery [102]. Molecular mechanisms behind ivosidenib resistance have been recently examined on 174 R/R AML patients included in a phase 1 dose-escalation and dose-expansion study (NCT02074839, Table 1) [103]. This study confirmed that mutations in RTK pathway genes are associated with a primary treatment resistance mechanism and are a frequent secondary resistance mechanism. *KRAS* mutations were more frequent at relapse or progression than at the start of treatment with ivosidenib. Second-site mutations in *IDH1* and mutations in *IDH2* are 2-HG-restoring mutations at relapse after complete remission and complete remission with partial hematologic recovery [103].

Enasidenib (AG-221, CC-90007)

Enasidenib is a first-in-class, an oral small-molecule, selective inhibitor of mutant IDH2 enzymes (Figure 6). In preclinical studies, enasidenib-induced inhibition of aberrant IDH2 protein decreased total serum 2-HG by more than 90%, reduced abnormal histone hypermethylation, and restored myeloid differentiation [104]. Enasidenib was also associated with a dose-dependent survival advantage in a primary AML xenotransplant model [104]. Enasidenib is not cytotoxic and acts as a differentiation agent. The first-in-human, phase 1/2 study assessed the maximum tolerated dose, safety, pharmacokinetic and pharmacodynamic profiles, and clinical activity of enasidenib in 176 patients with relapsed or refractory acute myeloid leukemia (NCT01915498, Table 2) [105]. The maximum tolerated dose was not reached at doses ranging from 50 to 650 mg per day. Enasidenib 100 mg once daily was selected for the expansion phase based on pharmacokinetic and pharmacodynamic profiles and demonstrated efficacy. The most common adverse events were hyperbilirubinemia (12%) and differentiation syndrome (7%). The overall response rate was 40.3%, median response duration of 5.8

months, and median overall survival was 9.3 months [105-107]. Huge reductions of 2-HG were found in almost all patients on enasidenib treatment, irrespective of clinical outcome. Thus, a reduction of 2-HG levels is not sufficient for clinical response. Similarly, *IDH2* mutational burden was not predictive, as responses were seen in patients with minor *IDH2* mutant subclones as well as in patients with fully clonal *IDH2* mutations [106]. A higher level of accompanying mutations and RAS pathway mutations were found in cases of non-responders.

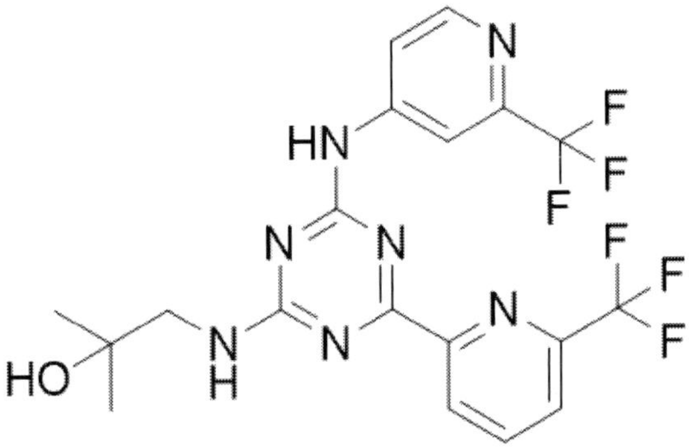

Figure 6. The chemical structure of enasidenib (AG-221). This small molecule functions as orally available inhibitor of mutated mitochondrial isocitrate dehydrogenase 2 (IDH2).

Ivosidenib or Enasidenib Combined with Intensive Treatment

The addition of cytotoxic therapy could reduce the risk of differentiation syndrome as an adverse event in enasidenib treatment and should also decrease the time to achieve complete remission in comparison with single-agent therapy. Ivosidenib or enasidenib combined with intensive chemotherapy in patients with newly diagnosed mutant *IDH1* or *IDH2* AML were studied in a phase 1 study [108, 109]. This clinical trial was registered as NCT02632708 (Table 2). Fit patients with AML undergoing first-line intensive 7 + 3 induction with intermediate- or high-dose cytarabine-based consolidation therapy were targeted with ivosidenib (500 mg per day) or enasidenib (100 mg per day) starting on day 1 of induction chemotherapy. A total of 60 patients were included in ivosidenib arm and 91 patients in enasidenib arm, respectively. Complete remission rate was 55% in the ivosidenib arm and the combined complete remission and complete remission with partial hematologic recovery was 72%. Complete remission rate was 47% in the enasidenib arm and the combined complete remission and complete remission with partial hematologic recovery was 62%. Comprehensive bone marrow biopsy review was done in 36 patients from this study [110]. Patients were categorized into 3 groups based on cellularity and blast composition on day 14 of therapy. The first group was aplasia (D14A) with <10% cellular and <5% blasts. The second group was differentiation (D14D) with >10% cellular and >5% blasts and with clearance of blasts at day 14 or day 21. The third group was persistent AML (D14P) with >10% cellular and >5% blasts and with no differentiation or clearance of blasts at day 14 or later. D14D was more common in patients receiving enasidenib (39%) than in patients receiving ivosidenib (20%) and was seen in 4 of 6 patients with an *IDH2*^{R172} mutation. *NPM1* and *RAS*-pathway co-mutations were relatively common in D14A patients but were rare in D14D patients. Induction chemotherapy has a high response rate in *NPM1*-mutated AML and induces *RAS*-pathway mutation clearance. D14A may represent leukemic clones that are rapidly eliminated by this combination therapy. On the other hand, D14D may reflect clones that differentiate by this combination therapy.

Ivosidenib or Enasidenib Combined with Azacitidine

Intensive chemotherapy regimens are often unsuitable for older patients or individuals with comorbidities. Hypomethylating agents (azacitidine, decitabine) can induce responses and prolong survival in patients ineligible for intensive chemotherapy. Because azacitidine and ivosidenib or enasidenib have a similar mechanism of action, their combination may confer additional clinical benefit over single-agent therapy. The enhanced cellular differentiation with combination treatment was shown by increased mRNA for hemoglobin F expression, and reduction of the $CD34^+$ cell population in the TF-1 cell model with IDH2^{R140Q} and also observed in primary samples from AML patients with IDH2 mutations [111]. In these primary samples treatment with a combination of enasidenib and azacitidine also reduced the immature CD34$^+$ cell population and increased the mature CD15$^+$ granulocyte/monocyte cell population. The randomized phase 2 part of study NCT02677922 (Table 2) evaluated the safety and efficacy of injectable azacitidine plus enasidenib in comparison to azacitidine alone in newly diagnosed AML patients with mutant IDH2. Preliminary data indicated that combination therapy significantly increased rates of response compared with azacitidine alone.

Table 2. Clinical trials with IDH2 inhibitors in adult AML and MDS with mutant *IDH2*

Trial Identification	Disease	Phase	Drugs
NCT03881735	*R/R AML*	2	enasidenib
NCT03683433	*R/R AML*	2	enasidenib plus azacitidine
NCT03825796	R/R AML	2	enasidenib plus CPX-351
NCT01915498	advanced AML	1/2	enasidenib
NCT03013998	previously untreated AML	1/2	enasidenib
NCT02632708	newly diagnosed AML	1	enasidenib plus standard chemotherapy
NCT02677922	newly diagnosed AML	1/2	enasidenib plus azacitidine
NCT03383575	high-risk MDS, R/R MDS	2	enasidenib plus azacitidine
NCT03839771	newly diagnosed AML	3	enasidenib plus standard chemotherapy
NCT03515512	post-HSCT AML	1	enasidenib as maintenance therapy after HSCT
NCT03728335	post-HSCT AML	1	enasidenib as maintenance therapy after HSCT
NCT02577406	AML >60 years	3	enasidenib versus conventional rare regimens

The overall response was 68% when the combination was used and 42% in the case of azacitidine alone [112]. Therefore, the inhibition of DNA methylation (writer DNMT) and reactivation of an eraser (TET) would lead to a release of a block on myeloid differentiation.

A preclinical study suggested that the addition of azacitidine to ivosidenib enhances mutant IDH1 inhibition-related differentiation and apoptosis. An open-label, multicenter, phase 1b trial evaluated the safety and efficacy of combining oral ivosidenib 500 mg once daily with subcutaneous azacitidine (75 mg/m^2 on days 1-7 in 28-day cycles in patients with newly diagnosed mutant *IDH1* AML) [113]. The overall response rate was 78.3% and complete remission was 60.9%. After a median follow-up of 16 months, the median overall survival was not reached with an estimated 1-year overall survival of 82%. Many patients with co-mutations (NRAS, KRAS, and PTPN11) with resistance to single-agent ivosidenib achieved remission with the combination of ivosidenib and azacitidine [113]. These promising results led to the current AGILE phase 3 trial (Table 1) [114]. The trial AGILE is a randomized study of azacitidine with or without ivosidenib in patients with newly diagnosed mutant *IDH1* AML not eligible for intensive chemotherapy [115]. The primary endpoint was changed from overall survival to event-free survival, defined as the time from randomization until treatment failure, relapse from remission, or death from any cause. Treatment failure is defined as non-fulfillment to achieve complete remission by week 24 [116].

Other Combinations Including IDH Inhibitors

A phase 1b/2 trial studied the safety, tolerability, and response rate of adding ivosidenib to either venetoclax alone, or to the combination of azacitidine plus venetoclax to treat AML patients with an *IDH1* mutation (Clinical Trial NCT03471260, Table 1) [117]. Eligible patients age ≥18 with *IDH1* mutated myeloid malignancies (high-risk MDS and AML) were enrolled into one of three successive cohorts (Cohort 1: ivosidenib+venetoclax 400 mg, Cohort 2: ivosidenib+venetoclax 800 mg, Cohort 3: ivosidenib+venetoclax 400 mg+AZA). Primary endpoints include safety and tolerability and overall response rate (ORR) by revised International Working Group (IWG) criteria. Key secondary endpoints include survival endpoints and pharmacokinetic correlates. 19 patients (median age 68) enrolled, 17 with AML: 9 relapsed/refractory AML (R/R; median 1 prior line of therapy), 5 treatment naïve AML, and 3 hypomethylating agents (HMA)-failure MDS with secondary AML. Two patients had high-risk MDS. European LeukemiaNet risk classification was favorable, intermediate, and adverse risk in 37%, 15%, and 47%. Co-mutations included *NPM1* (37%), chromatin-spliceosome (32%), methylation (16%), and RAS pathway (21%). Adverse events of special interest included IDH differentiation syndrome (n = 4, grade > 3 in 1) and tumor lysis syndrome (TLS; n = 2), including one grade 3 TLS event in an *NPM1$^+$* patient (successfully managed without hemodialysis). In evaluable patients (n = 18), composite complete remission (CRc: CR+CR$_i$+CR$_h$) rates were 78% overall (treatment-naive: 100%, R/R: 75%), and 67%, 100%, and 67% by cohort (median time to best response: 2 months). 7 (50%) patients achieving CRc were also minimal residual disease (MRD) negative by flow cytometry. The term CR$_i$ describes complete remission with incomplete count recovery and the term CR$_h$ describes marrow blast clearance and evidence of partial hematologic recovery. CR$_p$ is similar to CR$_i$, but specifically refers to the absence of platelet recovery [118]. 1 patient had hematologic improvement without CR/CR$_i$ and 1 had a morphological leukemia-free state. 9 (50%) patients remain on study, 3 (17%) proceeded to stem cell transplant in CR, 2 were non-responders, and 5 (22%) experienced progressive disease following CR$_c$ occurring after a median of 3 months. After a median follow-up of 3.5 months, median overall survival was not reached in treatment naïve patients, and 9.7 months in R/R patients. Ivosidenib+venetoclax+azacitidine therapy is well tolerated and highly effective for patients with *IDH1* mutated AML. Follow-up and an earned revenue evaluation are necessary procedures to better define duration and biomarkers of response [117].

Several studies showed that *IDH1* and *IDH2* mutations caused increased DNA damage, impaired homologous recombination, and increased sensitization to daunorubicin, irradiation, and the PARP inhibitors in cancer cells including AML cells [119-123]. Homologous recombination is also faulty in tumors carrying *BRCA1* or *BRCA2* mutations, which are vulnerable to PARP inhibitors like olaparib (Lynparza; AstraZeneca). Experiments were carried out to determine whether these drugs would also be effective in *IDH*-mutant tumors. Researchers found that olaparib and other PARP inhibitors killed cells in multiple cancer cell lines that harbor *IDH1* and *IDH2* mutations. In addition, glioma cell lines generated from patient tumors with *IDH1* mutations were vulnerable to the investigational PARP inhibitor talazoparib (BMN-673; Medivation). In mice, olaparib slowed the growth of implanted *IDH1*-mutant tumors. The findings suggested that any tumor with *IDH* mutations will likely be susceptible to PARP inhibitors. However, accompanying administration of selective inhibitors of mutant IDH1 and IDH2 enzymes during cytotoxic therapy decrease the efficacy of both PARP inhibitors and IDH inhibitors [119].

VACCINATION AS PROMISING THERAPEUTIC APPROACH FOR THE MUTANT *IDH1* AND *IDH2*-DIVEN MALIGNANCIES

Platten et al. recently described a new vaccination strategy targeting the major histocompatibility complex (MHC) class II-associated IDH1^{R132H} neoepitope peptide in adult patients with gliomas carrying this mutation [124, 125]. Preclinical studies showed that IDH1^{R132H} vaccination induced specific T helper immune responses associated with therapeutic benefit in syngeneic, MHC-humanized mice [126]. There were no dose-limiting toxicities in a clinical trial, where 29 of the 32 patients with newly diagnosed IDH1^{R132H} WHO grade 3 or 4 glial tumors completed all planned study vaccinations. The rate of vaccine-induced systemic immune responses was striking and irrespective of HLA type. Among 30 patients, peripheral T cell and humoral B cell immune responses specific to IDH1^{R132H} were found in 26 (87%) and 28 (93%) patients, respectively [124]. This approach offers powerful therapeutic promise for all mutant *IDH*-driven cancers.

CONCLUSION

Recurrent somatic mutations in the genes encoding for IDH1 and IDH2 were detected in about 20% of patients with AML and 5% of patients with MDS. Mutations in IDH1 or IDH2 enzymes affect their enzymatic activity making them able to convert α-ketoglutarate to 2-hydroxyglutarate and competitively inhibit α-ketoglutarate-dependent enzymes, alter DNA and histone methylation, and impair cellular growth and differentiation. The availability of IDH inhibitors, besides the development of other targeted drugs, such as FLT3 inhibitors, venetoclax, and others, represents great progress in AML therapy. For decades, the standard induction for patients with acute myeloid leukemia (AML) has been the combination of cytarabine with anthracycline (7 + 3 regimen). In August 2017, the US FDA approved CPX-351 (vyxeos), a liposomal formulation of cytarabine and daunorubicin at a fixed 5:1 molar ratio, for the treatment of adults with newly diagnosed AML with myelodysplasia-related changes (AML-MRC) and therapy-related AML (t-AML). This is the first approved treatment specifically for patients with this subgroup of AML.

A prognostic significance of concurrent gene mutations in intensively treated patients with *IDH*-mutated AML was studied in ALFA trials [127]. The associations with other mutations were studied in the two most frequent mutant *IDH1* variants (*IDH1* R132H and *IDH1* R132C) and mutant *IDH2* variants (*IDH2* R140 and *IDH2* R172). Mutant IDH1^{R132H} enzyme was present in younger patients (median age, 56 years versus 63 years for other IDH1 variants) and is associated with higher white blood cell counts. This variant was more associated with *NPM1* mutations and with *FLT3-ITD* than other IDH1 variants (64% vs 34%; 27% vs 6%). Mutant IDH1^{R132C} enzyme had higher rates of trisomy 8 (23% vs 5% for other IDH1 variants), as well as mutations in *PHF6* (gene coding homeodomain PHD finger protein 6), *BCOR* (gene coding BCL6 corepressor), and *BCORL1* (gene coding BCL6 corepressor like 1). Despite these two diverse mutational patterns, there was no difference in survival between patients with IDH1^{R132H} or IDH1^{R132C}. Mutant IDH2^{R140} variants were associated with higher rates of *NPM1* mutations and *FLT3-ITD*, *SRSF2* splicing mutation, normal karyotype, and higher white blood cell counts. *NPM1* mutations predicted prolonged overall survival and disease-free survival. *DNMT3A* mutations had the opposite effect. Patients with mutant IDH2^{R172} had lower white blood cell counts, more frequent *BCOR* mutations, and no *NPM1* mutations. *NPM1* was the only mutation predicting overall survival for patients with mutant *IDH1* and mutant *IDH2* R140. Other mutations including *FLT3-ITD* had no significant prognostic impact. Future clinical trials testing frontline IDH inhibitors combined with intensive chemotherapy should consider stratification on *NPM1* mutational status. Allogeneic hematopoietic stem cell transplantation improved the overall survival of unfavorable *IDH*-mutated AML and should be integrated into the treatment strategy [127].

Whether it is useful to incorporate enasidenib or ivosidenib in the azacitidine plus venetoclax combination, that is changing the standard of care for older newly diagnosed AML patients, should be necessary for a study about higher benefit given by azacitidine plus venetoclax in *IDH*-mutated AML [111-117].

ACKNOWLEDGMENTS

This work was supported by the project for conceptual development of research organization No 00023736 (Institute of Hematology and Blood Transfusion) from the Ministry of Health of the Czech Republic.

REFERENCES

[1] Parsons, DW; Jones, S; Zhang, X; Lin, JC; Leary, RJ; Angenendt, P; et al. An integrated genomic analysis of human glioblastoma multiforme. *Science.*, 2008, 321, 1807-1812.

[2] Yan, H; Parsons, DW; Jin, G; McLendon, R; Rasheed, BA; Yuan, W; et al. IDH1 and IDH2 mutations in gliomas. *N. Engl. J. Med.*, 2009, 360, 765-773.

[3] Han, S; Liu, Y; Cai, SJ; Qian, M; Ding, J; Larion, M; et al. IDH mutation in glioma: molecular mechanisms and potential therapeutic targets. *Br. J. Cancer.*, 2020, 122, 1580-1589.

[4] Mardis, ER; Ding, L; Dooling, DJ; Larson, DE; McLellan, MD; Chen, K; et al. Recurring mutations found by sequencing an acute myeloid leukemia genome. *N. Engl. J. Med.*, 2009, 361, 1058-1066.

[5] Kipp, BR; Voss, JS; Kerr, SE; Barr Fritcher, EG; Graham, RP; Zhang, L; et al. Isocitrate dehydrogenase 1 and 2 mutations in cholangiocarcinoma. *Hum. Pathol.*, 2012, 43, 1552-1558.

[6] Amary, MF; Bacsi, K; Maggiani, F; Damato, S; Halai, D; Berisha, F; et al. IDH1 and IDH2 mutations are frequent events in central chondrosarcoma and central and periosteal chondromas but not in other mesenchymal tumours. *J. Pathol.*, 2011, 224, 334-343.

[7] Atai, NA; Renkema-Mills, NA; Bosman, J; Schmidt, N; Rijkeboer, D; Tigchelaar, W; et al. Differential activity of NASPH-producing dehydrogenases renders rodents ubsuitable models to study IDH1R132 mutation effects in human glioblastoma. *J. Histochem. Cytochem.*, 2011, 59, 489-503.

[8] Chatuvedi, A; Araujo Cruz, MM; Jyotsama, N; Sharma, A; Yu, TH; Görlich, K; et al. Mutant IDH1 promotes leukemogenesis *in vivo* and can be specifically targeted in human AML. *Blood.*, 2013, 122, 2877-2887.

[9] Badur, MG; Muthusamy, T; Parker, SJ; Ma, S; McBrayer, SK; Cordes, T; et al. Oncogenic R132IDH1 mutationslimit NADPH for *de novo* lipogenesis through (D)2-hydroxyglutarate production in fibrosarcoma cells. *Cell. Rep.*, 2018, 25, 1018.e4-1026.e4.

[10] Salati, M; Caputo, F; Baldessari, C; Galasi, B; Grossi, F; Dominici, M; Ghidini, M. IDH signalling pathway in cholangiocarcinoma: From biological rationale to therapeutic targeting. *Cancers* (Basel)., 2020, 12, 3310.

[11] Dalziel, K. Isocitrate dehydrogenase and related oxidative decarboxylases. *FEBS Lett.*, 1980, 117, K45-K55.

[12] Waitkus, MS; Diplas, BH; Yan, H. Isocitrate dehydrugenase mutations in gliomas. *Neuro. Oncol.*, 2016, 18, 16-26.

[13] Medeiros, BC; Fathi, AT; DiNardo, CD; Pollyea, DA; Chan, SM; Swords, R. Isocitrate dehydrogenase mutations in myeloid malignancies. *Leukemia.*, 2017, 31, 272-281.

[14] Dang, L; White, DW; Gross, S; Bennett, BD; Bittinger, MA; Driggers, EM; et al. Cancer associated IDH1 mutations produce 2-hydroxyglutarate. *Nature.*, 2009, 462, 739-744.
[15] Gross, S; Caims, RA; Minden, MD; Driggers, EM; Bittinger, MA; Jang, HG; et al. Cancer-associated metabolite 2-hydroxyglutarate accumulates in acute myelogenous leukemia with isocitrate dehydrogenase 1 and 2 mutations. *J. Exp. Med.*, 2010, 207, 339-344.
[16] Ward, PS; Patel, J; Wise, DR; Abdel-Wahab, O; Bennett, BD; Coller, HA; et al. The common feature of leukemia-associated IDH1 and IDH2 mutations is a neomorphic enzyme activity converting α-ketoglutarate to 2-hydroxyglutarate. *Cancer Cell.*, 2010, 17, 225-234.
[17] Ye, D; Guan, KL; Xiong, Y. Metabolism, activity, and targeting of D- and L-2-hydroxyglutarates. *Trends Cancer.*, 2018, 4, 151-165.
[18] Dang, L; Su, SM. Isocitrate dehydrogenase mutation and (R)-2-hydroxyglutarate: From basic discovery to therapeutics development. *Annu. Rev. Biochem.*, 2017, 86, 305-331.
[19] Narahara, K; Kimura, S; Kikkawa, K; Takahashi, Y; Wakita, Y; Kasai, R; et al. Probable assignment of soluble isocitrate dehydrogenase (IDH1) to 2q33.3. *Hum. Genet.*, 1985, 71, 37–40.
[20] Al-Khallaf, H. Isocitrate dehydrogenases in physiology and cancer: biochemical and molecular insight. *Cell Biosci.*, 2017, 7, 37.
[21] Stoddard, BL; Dean, A; Koshland, DE; Jr. Structure of isocitrate dehydrogenase with isocitrate, nicotinamide adenine dinucleotide phosphate, and calcium at 2.5-A resolution: a pseudo-Michaelis ternary complex. *Biochemistry.*, 1993, 32, 9310-9316.
[22] Testa, U; Castelli, G; Pelosi, E. Isocitrate dehydrogenase mutation in myelodysplastic syndromes and in acute myeloid leukemias. *Cancers.*, 2020; 12, 2427.
[23] Xu, X; Zhao, J; Xu, Z; Peng, B; Huang, Q; Arnold, E; Ding, J. Structures of human cytosolic NADP-dependent isocitrate dehydrogenase revealed a novel self-regulatory mechanism of activity. *J. Biol. Chem.*, 2004, 279, 33946-33957.
[24] Tommasini-Ghelfi, S; Murnan, K; Kouri, FM; Mahajan, AS; May, JL; Stegh AH. Cancer-associated mutation and beyond: The

emerging biology of isocitrate dehydrogenases in human disease. *Sci. Adv.*, 2019, 5, eaaw4543.

[25] Xu, Y; Liu, L; Nakamura, A; Someya, S; Miyakawa, T; Tanokura, M. Studies on the regulatory mechanism of isocitrate dehydrogenase 2 using acetylation mimics. *Sci. Rep.*, 2017, 7, 9785.

[26] Sun, P; Ma, T; Zhang, T; Zhu, H; Zhang, J; Liu, Y; Ding, J. Molecular basis for the function of the heterodimer of human NAD-dependent isocitrate dehydrogenase. *J. Biol. Chem,.* 2019, 294, 16214-16227.

[27] Cairns, RA; Mak, TW. Oncogenic isocitrate dehydrogenase mutation: mechanisms, models, and clinical opportunities. *Cancer Discov.* 2013, 3, 730-741.

[28] Smolková, K; Špačková, J; Gotvaldová, K; Dvořák, A; Křenková, A; Hubálek, M; et al. SIRT3 and GCN5L regulation of $NADP^+$- and NADPH-driven reactions of mitochondrial isocitrate dehydrogenase IDH2. *Sci. Rep.*, 2020, 10, 8677.

[29] Losman, JA; Kaelin, WG. Jr. What a difference a hydroxyl makes: mutant IDH, (R)-2-hydroxyglutarate, and cancer. *Genes Dev.*, 2013, 27, 836-852.

[30] Kranendijk, M; Struys, EA; Salomons, GS; Van der Knaap, MS; Jakobs, C. Progress in understanding 2-hydroxyglutaric acidurias. *J. Inherit. Metab. Dis.*, 2012, 35, 571-587.

[31] Du, X; Hu, H. The roles of 2-hydroxyglutarate. *Front. Cell Develop. Biol.*, 2021, 9, article 651317.

[32] Choi, C; Ganji, SK; DeBerardinis, RJ; Hatanpaa, KJ; Rakheja, D; Kovacs, Z; et al. 2-hydroxyglutarate detection by magnetic resonance spectroscopy in IDH-mutated patients with gliomas. *Nat. Med.*, 2012, 18, 624-629.

[33] Chowdhury, R; Yeoh, KK; Tian, YM; Hillringhaus, L; Bagg, EA; Rose, NR; et al. The oncometabolite 2-hydroxyglutarate inhibits histone lysine demethylases. *EMBO Rep.*, 2011, 12, 463-469.

[34] Xu, W; Yang, H; Liu, Y; Yang, Y; Wang, P; Kim, SH; et al. Oncometabolite 2-hydroxyglutarate is a competitive inhibitor of α-ketoglutarate-dependent dioxygenases. *Cancer Cell.*, 2011, 19, 17-30.

[35] Koivunen, P; Lee, S; Duncan, CG; Lopez, G; Lu, G; Ramkissoon, S; et al. Transformation by the (R)-enantiomer of 2-hydroxyglutarate linked to EGLN activation. *Nature.*, 2012, 483, 484-488.

[36] Lu, C; Ward, PS; Kapoor, GS; Rohle, D; Turcan, S; Abdel-Wahab, O; et al. IDH mutation impairs histone demethylation and results in a block to cell differentiation. *Nature.*, 2012, 483, 474-478.

[37] McBrayer, SK; Mayers, JR; DiNatale, GJ; Shi, DD; Khanai, J; Chakraborty, AA; et al. Transaminase inhibition by 2-hydroxyglutarate impairs glutamate biosynthesis and redox homeostasis in glioma. *Cell.*, 2018, 175, 101-116 e125.

[38] Tateishi, K; Wakimoto, H; Iafrate, AJ; Tanaka, S; Loebel, F; Lelic, N; et al. Extreme vulnerability of IDH1 mutant cancers to NAD$^+$ depletion. *Cancer Cell.*, 2015, 28, 773-784.

[39] Dan, Y; Xiong, Y; Guan, GL. The mechanism of IDH mutations in tumorigenesis. *Cell Res.*, 2012, 22, 1102-1104.

[40] Nassereddine, S; Lap, CJ; Haroun, F; Tabbara, I. The role of mutant IDH1 and IDH2 inhibitors in the treatment of acute myeloid leukemia. *Ann. Hematol.*, 2017, 96, 1983-1991.

[41] Figueroa, ME; Abdel-Wahab, O; Lu, C; Ward, PS; Patel, J; Shih, A; et al. Leukemic IDH1 and IDH2 mutations result in a hypermethylation phenotype, disrupt TET2 function, and impair hematopoietic differentiation. *Cancer Cell.*, 2010, 18, 553-567.

[42] Kernytsky, A; Wang, F; Hansen, E; Schalm, S; Straley, K; Gliser, C; et al. IDH2 mutation-induced histone and DNA hypermethylation is progressively reversed by small–molecule inhibition. *Blood.*, 2015, 125, 296-303.

[43] Wang, F; Travins, J; DeLaBarre, B; Pernard-Lacronique, V; Schalm, C; Hansen, E; et al. Taargeted inhibition of mutant IDH2 in leukemic cells induces cellular differentiation. *Science.*, 2013, 340, 622-626.

[44] Chan, SM; Thomas, D; Corces-Zimmerman, MR; Xavy, S; Rastogi, S; Hong, WJ; et al. Isocitrate dehydrogenase 1 and 2 mutations induce BCL-2 dependence in acute myeloid leukemia. *Nat. Med.*, 2015, 21, 178-184.

[45] Gu, Y; Yang, R; Yang, Y; Zhao, Y; Wakeham, A; Wanda, YL; et al. *IDH1* mutation contributes to myeloid dysplasia in mice by

disturbing heme biosynthesis and erythropoiesis. *Blood.*, 2021, 137, 945-958.

[46] Sasaki, M; Knobbe, CB; Munger, JC; Lind, EF; Brenner, D; Brüstle, A; et al. IDH1(R132H) mutation increases murine haematopoietic progenitors and alters epigenetics. *Nature.*, 2012, 488, 656-659.

[47] Inoue, S; Li, WY; Tseng, A; Beerman, I; Elia, AJ; Bendall, SC; et al. Mutant IDH1 downregulates ATM and alters DNA repair and sensitivity to DNA damage independent of TET2. *Cancer Cell.*, 2016, 30, 337-348.

[48] Qing, Z; Dong, L; Gao, L; Li, C; Li, Y; Han, L; et al. R-2-hydroxyglutarate attenuates aerobic glycolysis in leukemia by targeting the FTO/m^{6}A/PFKP/LDHB axis. *Mol. Cell.*, 2021, 81, 922-939 e9.

[49] Su, R; Dong, L; Li, C; Nachtergaele, S; Wunderlich, M; Qing, Y; et al. R-2HG exhibits anti-tumor activity by targeting FTO/m^{6}A/MYC/CEBPA signaling. *Cell.*, 2018, 172, 90-105 e23.

[50] Jaiswal, S; Fontanillas, P; Flannick, J; Manning, A; Grauman, PV; Mar, BG; et al. Age-related clonal hematopoiesis associated with adverse outcomes. *N. Engl. J. Med.*, 2014, 371, 2488-2498.

[51] Jan, M; Ebert, BL; Jaiswal, S. Clonal hematopoiesis. *Semin. Hematol.*, 2017, 54, 43-50.

[52] Shlush, LI. Age-related clonal hematopoiesis. *Blood.*, 2018, 131, 496-504.

[53] Jaiswal, S; Ebert, BL. Clonal hematopoiesis in human aging and disease. *Science.*, 2019, 366, eaan4673.

[54] Desai, P; Mencia-Trinchant, M; Savenkov, O; Simon, MS; Cheang, G; Lee, S; et al. Somatic mutations precede acute myeloid leukemia years before diagnosis. *Nat. Med.*, 2018, 24, 1015-1023.

[55] Bowman, RL; Busque, L; Levine, RL. Clonal hematopoiesis and evaluation to hematopoietic malignancies. *Cell Stem Cell.*, 2018, 22, 157-170.

[56] Bejar, R; Steensma, DP. Recent developments in myelodysplastic syndromes. *Blood.*, 2014, 124, 2793-2803.

[57] Pellagatti, A; Boultwood, J. The molecular pathogenesis of the myelodysplastic syndromes. *Eur. J. Haematol.*, 2015, 95, 3-15.

[58] Shastri, A; Will, B; Steidl, U; Verma, A. Stem and progenitor cell alterations in myelodysplastic syndromes. *Blood.*, 2017, 129, 1586-1594.
[59] Nazha, A; Sekeres, MA. Precision medicine in myelodysplastic syndromes and leukemias: Lessons from sequential mutations. *Annu. Rev. Med.*, 2017, 68, 127-137.
[60] Nazha, A. The MDS genomics-prognosis symbiosis. *Hematology. American Society of Hematology Education Program.*, 2018, 2018, 270-276.
[61] Barreyro, L; Chlon, TM; Starczynowski, DT. Chronic immune response dysregulation in MDS pathogenesis. *Blood.*, 2018, 132, 1553-1560.
[62] Papaemmanuil, E; Gerstung, M; Malcovati, L; Tauro, S; Gundem, G; Van Loo, P; et al. Clinical and biological implications of driver mutations in myelodysplastic syndromes. *Blood.*, 2013, 122, 3616-3627.
[63] Haferlach, T; Nagata, Y; Grossmann, V; Okuno, Y; Bacher, U; Nagwe, G; et al. Landscape of genetic lesions in 944 patients with myelodysplastic syndromes. *Leukemia.*, 2014, 28, 241-247.
[64] Molenaar, RJ; Thota, S; Nagata, Y; Patel, B; Clemente, M; Hirsh, C; et al. Clinical and biological implications of ancestral and non-ancestral IDH1 and IDH2 mutations in myeloid neoplasms. *Leukemia.*, 2015, 29, 2134-2142.
[65] DiNardo, C; Jabbour, E; Ravandi, F; Takahashi, K; Daver, N; Routbort, M; et al. IDH1 and IDH2 mutations in myelodysplastic syndromes and role in disease progression. *Leukemia.*, 2016, 30, 980-984.
[66] Marcucci, G; Maharry, K; Wu, YZ; Radmacher, MD; Mrózek, K; Margeson, D; et al. *IDH1* and *IDH2* gene mutations identify novel molecular subsets within de novo cytogenetically normal acute myeloid leukemia: a cancer and leukemia group B study. *J. Clin. Oncol.*, 2010, 28, 2348-2355.
[67] Lin, TL; Nagata, Y; Kao, HW; Sanada, M; Okuno, Y; Huang, CF; et al. Clonal leukemic evolution in myelodysplastic syndromes with TET2 and IDH1-IDH2 mutations. *Haematologica.*, 2014, 99, 28-36.

[68] Makishima, H; Yoshizato, T; Yoshida, K; Sekeres, MA; Radivoyevitch, T; Suzuki, H; et al. Dynamics of clonal evolution in myelodysplastic syndromes. *Nat. Genet.*, 2017, 49, 204-212.

[69] Chou, WC; Lei, WC; Ko, BS; Hou, HA; Chen, CY; Tang, JL; et al. The prognostic impact and stability of isocitrate dehydrogenase 2 mutation in adult patients with acute myeloid leukemia. *Leukemia.*, 2011, 25, 246-253.

[70] Patel, JP; Gönen, M; Figueroa, ME; Fernandez, H; Sun, Z; Racevskis, J; et al. Prognostic relevance of integrated genetic profiling in acute myeloid leukemia. *N. Engl. J. Med.*, 2012, 366, 1079-1089.

[71] Green, CL; Evans, CM; Zhao, L; Hills, RK; Burnett, AK; Linch, DC; Gale, RE. The prognostic significance of IDH2 mutations in AML depends on the location of the mutation. *Blood.*, 2010, 118, 409-412.

[72] Zarnegar-Lumley, S; Alonzo, TA; Othus, M; Sun, Z; Ries, RE; Wang, YC; et al. Characteristics and Prognostic Effects of IDH Mutations Across the Age Spectrum in AML: A Collaborative Analysis from COG; SWOG; and ECOG. Presented at: 62nd American Society of Hematology Annual Meeting & Exposition; December 5-8; 2020. Abstract 388. *Blood.*, 2020, 136(Suppl.1), 31-32.

[73] Duchmann, M; Micol, JB; Duployez, N; Raffoux, E; Thomas, X; Marolleau, JP; et al. Prognostic significance of concurrent gene mutations in intensively treated patients with IDH 1/2 mutated AML. *Blood.*, 2021, doi, 10.1182/blood. 2020010165.

[74] Thol, F; Damm, F; Wagner, K; Göhring, G; Schlegelberger, B; Hoelzer, D; et al. Prognostic impact of IDH2 mutations in cytogenetically normal acute myeloid leukemia. *Blood.*, 2020, 116, 614-616.

[75] Ravandi, F; Patel, K; Luthra, R; Faderl, S; Konopleva, M; Kadia, T; et al. Prognostic significance of alterations in IDH enzyme isoforms in patients with AML treated with high-dose cytarabine and idarubicin. *Cancer.*, 118, 2665-2673.

[76] Boissel, N; Nibourel, O; Renneville, A; Gardin, C; Reman, O; Contentin, N; et al. Prognostic impact of isocitrate dehydrogenase enzyme isoforms 1 and 2 mutations in acute myeloid leukemia: a

study by the Acute Leukemia French Association group. *J. Clin. Oncol.*, 2010, 28, 3717-3723.

[77] Paschka, P; Schlenk, RF; Gaizdik, RF; Habdank, M; Krönke, J; Bullinger, L; et al. IDH1 and IDH2 mutations are frequent genetic alterations in acute myeloid leukemia and confer adverse prognosis in cytogenetically normal acute myeloid leukemia with NPM1 mutation without FLT3 pnternal tandem duplication. *J. Clin. Oncol.*, 2010, 28, 3636-3643.

[78] DiNardo, CD; Ravandi, F; Agresta, S; Konopleva, M; Takahashi, K; Kadia, T; et al. Characteristics, clinical outcome, and prognostic significance of IDH mutations in AML. *Am. J. Hematol.*, 2015, 90, 732-736.

[79] Yamaguchi, S; Iwanaga, E; Tokunaga, K; Nanri, T; Shimomura, T; Suzushima, H; et al. IDH1 and IDH2 mutations confer an adverse effect in patients with acute myeloid leukemia lacking the NPM1 mutation. *Eur. J. Haematol.*, 2014, 62, 471-477.

[80] Pardanani, A; Lasho, TL; Finke, CM; Mai, M; McClure, RF; Tefferi, A. IDH1 and IDH2 mutation analysis in chronic- and blast-phase myeloproliferative neoplasms. *Leukemia.*, 2010, 24, 1146-1151.

[81] Tefferi, A; Lasho, TL; Abdel-Wahab, O; Guglielmelli, P; Patel, J; Caramazza, D; et al. *Leukemia.*, 2010, 24, 1302-1309.

[82] Debarri, H; Lebon, D; Roumier, C; Check, M; Marceau-Renaut, A; Nibourel, D; et al. IDH1/IDH2 but not DNMT3A mutations are suitable targets for minimal residual disease monitoring in acute myeloid leukemia patient: A study in the Acute Leukemia French Association. *Oncotarget.*, 2015, 6, 42345-42353.

[83] Ok, CY; Loghavi, S; Sui, D; Wei, P; Kanagal-Shamanna, R; Yin, CC; et al. Persistent *IDH1/IDH2* mutations in remission can predict relapse in patients with acute myeloid leukemia. *Haematologica.*, 2019, 104, 305-311.

[84] Brambati, C; Galbiati, S; Xue, E; Toffalori, C; Crucitti, L; Greco, R; et al. Droplet digital polymerase chain reaction for DNMT3A a nd IDH1/IDH2 mutations to improve early detection of acute myeloid leukemia relapseter allogeneic hewmatopoietic stem cell transplantation. *Haematologica.*, 2016, 101, 305-311.

[85] Kattih, B; Shirvani, A; Klement, P; Garrido, AM; Gabdoulline, R; Liebich, A; et al. *IDH1/2* mutations in acute myeloid leukemia patients and risk of coronary artery disease and cardiac dysfunction–a retrospective propensity score analysis. *Leukemia.*, 2021, 35, 1301-1316.

[86] Chaturvedi, A; Herbst, L; Pusch, S; Klett, L; Goparaju, R; Stichel, D; et al. Pan-mutant IGH1 inhibitor BAY1436032 is highly effective against human IDH1 mutant acute myeloid leukemia *in vivo. Leukemia.*, 2017, 31, 2020-2028.

[87] Chaturvedi, A; Gupta, C; Gabdoulline, R; Borchert, NM; Goparaju, R; Kaulfuss, S; et al. Synergistic activity of IDH1 inhibitor BAY1436032 with azacitidine in IDH1 mutant acute myeloid leukemia. *Haematologica.*, 2021, 106, 565-573.

[88] Zeng, Z; Konopleva, M. Concurrent inhibition of IHD and methyltransferase maximizes therapeutic efficacy in IDH mutant acute myeloid leukemia. *Haematologica.*, 2021, 106, 324-326.

[89] Heuser, M; Palmisiano, N; Mantzaris, I; Mims, A; DiNardo, C; Silverman, LR; et al. Safety and efficacy of BAY1436032 in IDH1-mutant AML: phase 1 study results. *Leukemia.*, 2020, 34, 2903-2913.

[90] Caravella, JA; Lin, J; Diebold, RB; Campbell, AM; Ericsson, A; Gustafson, G; et al. Structure-based design and identification of FT-2102 (Olutasidenib); a potent mutant-selective IDH1 inhibitor. *J. Med. Chem.*, 2020, 63, 1612-1623.

[91] Watts, JM; Baer, MR; Yang, J; Prebet, T; Lee, S; Schiller, GJ; et al. Olutasidenib (FT-2102), an IDH1m inhibitor as a single agent or in combination with azacitidine, induces deep clinical responses with mutation clearance in patients treated in a phase 1 dose escalation and expansion study. *Blood.*, 2019, 134(Suppl. 1), 231.

[92] Cortes, JE; Wang, ES; Watts, JM; Lee, S; Baer, MR; Dao, KH; et al. Olutasidenib (FT-2102) induces rapid remissions in patients with IDH1-mutant myelodysplastic syndrome: results of phase 1/2 single agent treatment and combination with azacitidine. *Blood.*, 2019, 134(Suppl. 1), 674.

[93] DiNardo, CD; Schimmer, AD; Yee, KWL; Hochhaus, A; Kraemer, A; Carvajal, RD; et al. A pase I study of IDH305 in patients with

advanced malignancies including relapsed/refractory AML and MDS that harbor IDH1^{R132} mutations. *Blood.*, 2016, 128(22),1073.

[94] Cho, YS; Levell, JR; Liu, G; Caferro, T; Sutton, J; Shafer, CM; et al. Discovery and evaluation of clinical candidate IDH305, a brain penetrant mutant IDH1 inhibitor. *ACS Med. Chem. Lett.*, 2017, 8, 1116-1121.

[95] Popovici-Muller, J; Saunders, JO; Salituro, FG; Travins, J; Yan, S; Zhao, F; et al. Discovery of the first potent inhibitors of mutant IDH1 that lower tumor 2-HG *in vivo*. *ACS Med. Chem. Lett.*, 2012, 3, 850-855.

[96] Popovici-Muller, J; Lemieux, RM; Artin, E; Saunders, JO; Salituro, FG; Travins, J; et al. Discovery of AG-120 (Ivosidenib): a first-in-class mutant IDH1 inhibitor for the treatment of IDH1 mutant cancers. *ACS Med. Chem. Lett.*, 2018, 9, 300-305.

[97] Norsworthy, KJ; Luo, I; Hsu, V; Gudi, R; Dorff, SE; Przepiorka, D; et al. FDA Approval Summary: Ivosidenib for relapsed or refractory acute myeloid leukemia with an isocitrate dehydrogenase-1 mutation. *Clin. Cancer. Res.*, 2019, 25, 3205-3209.

[98] Dhillon, S. Ivosidenib: first global approval. *Drugs*, 2018, 78, 1509-1516.

[99] Pasquier, F; Lecuit, M; Broutin, S; Saada, S; Jeanson, A; Penard-Lacronique, V; et al. Ivosidenib to treat adult patients with relapsed or refractory acute myeloid leukemia. *Drugs Today (Barc).*, 2020, b56, 21-32.

[100] Cerchione, C; Romano, A; Daver, N; DiNardo, C; Jabbour, EJ; Konopleva, M; et al. IDH1/IDH2 inhibition in acute myeloid leukemia. *Front. Oncol.*, 2021, 11, 639387.

[101] DiNardo, CD; Stein, EM; de Botton, S; Roboz, GJ; Altman, JK; Mims, AS; et al. Durable remissions with ivosidenib in *IDH1*-mutated relapsed or refractory AML. *N. Engl. J. Med.*, 2018, 378, 2386-2398.

[102] Roboz, GJ; DiNardo, CD; Stein, EM; de Botton, S; Mims, AS; Prince, GT; et al. Ivosidenib induces deep durable remissions in patients with newly diagnosed *IDH1*-mutant acute myeloid leukemia. *Blood.*, 2020, 135, 463-471.

[103] Choe, S; Wang, H; DiNardo, CD; Stein, EM; de Botton, S; Roboz, GJ; et al. Molecular mechanisms mediating relapse following ivosidenib monotherapy in *IDH1*-mutant relapsed or refractory AML. *Blood Adv.*, 2020, 4, 1894-1905.
[104] Yen, K; Travins, J; Wang, F; David, MD; Artin, E; Straley, K; et al. AG-221, a first-in-class therapy targeting acute myeloid leukemia harboring oncogenic IDH2 mutations. *Cancer Discov.*, 2017, 7, 478-493.
[105] Stein, EM; DiNardo, CD; Pollyea, D; Fathi, AT; Roboz, GJ; Altman, KJ; et al. Enasidenib in mutant *IDH2* relapsed or refractory acute myeloid leukemia. *Blood.*, 2017, 130, 722-731.
[106] Amatangelo, MD; Quek, L; Shih, A; Stein, EM; Roshal, M; David, MD; et al. Enasidenib induces acute myeloid leukemia cell differentiation to promote clinical response. *Blood.*, 2017, 130, 732-741.
[107] Wouters, BJ. Hitting the target in *IDH2* mutant AML. *Blood.*, 2017, 130, 693-694.
[108] Stein, EM; DiNardo, CD; Fathi, AT; Mims, AS; Pratz, KW; Savona, MR; et al. Ivosidenib or enasidenib combined with intensive chemotherapy in patients with newly diagnosed AML: a phase 1 study. *Blood.*, 2021, 137, 1792-1803.
[109] Wei, AH; Daver, N. Taking aim at IDH in fitter patients with AML. *Blood.*, 2021, 137, 1706-1707.
[110] Mason, EF; Pozdnyakova, O; Roshal, M; Fathi, AT; Stein, AM; Ferrell, PB; et al. A novel differentiation response with combination IDH inhibitor and intensive induction therapy for AML. *Blood Adv.*, 2021, 5, 2279-2283.
[111] MacBeth, KJ; Chopra, VS; Tang, L; Zheng, B; Avanzino, B; See, WL; et al. Combination of azacitidine and enasidenib enhances leukemic cell differentiation and cooperatively hypomethylates DNA. *Exp. Hematol.*, 2021, doi, 10.1016/j.exphem.2021.03.003.
[112] DiNardo, CD; Schuh, AC; Stein, EM; Fernandez, PM; Wei, A; de Botton, S; et al. Enasidenib plus azacitidine significantly improves complete remission and overall response compared with azacitidine alone in patients with newly diagnosed acute myeloid leukemia (AML) with isocitrate dehydrogenase 2 (IDH2)

mutations: interim phase II results from an ongoing, randomized study. *Blood.*, 2019, 134(Suppl. 1), 643.

[113] DiNardo, CD; Stein, AS; Stein, EM; Fathi, AT; Frankfurt, O; Schuh, AC; et al. Mutant isocitrate dehydrogenase 1 inhibitor ivosidenib in combination with azacitidine for newly diagnosed acute myeloid leukemia. *J. Clin. Oncol.*, 2020, 39, 57-65.

[114] Fernandez, PM; Recher, C; Doronin, V; Calado, RT; Jang, JT; Miyasaki, Y; et al. A phase 3, multicenter, double-blind, randomized, placebo-controlled study of ivosidenib in combination with azacitidine in adult patients with previously untreated acute myeloid leukemia with an IDH1 mutation. *Blood.*, 2019, 134(Suppl. 1), 2593.

[115] Dragani, M; de Botton, S. SOHO state of the art updates and next questions: IDH inhibition. *Clin Lymphoma Myeloma Leuk.*, 2021, doi: 10.1016/j.clml.2021.05.004.

[116] Martelli, MP; Martino, G; Cardinali, V; Falini, B; Martinelli, G; Cerchione, C. Enasidenib and ivosidenib in AML. *Minerva Med.*, 2020, 111, 411-426.

[117] Lachowiez, CA; Borthakur, G; Loghavi, S; Zeng, Z; Kadia, TM; Masarova, L; et al. Phase Ib/II study of the IDH1-mutant inhibitor ivosidenib with the BCL2 inhibitor venetoclax +/- azacitidine in IDH1-mutated hematologic malignancies. *J. Clin. Oncol.*, 2020, 38, 7500.

[118] Shallis, RM; Pollyea, DA; Zeidan, AM. Complete, yet partial: the benefits of complete response with partial haematological recovery as an endpoint in acute myeloid leukaemia clinical trials. *Lancet Haematol.*, 2020, 7, 853-856.

[119] Molenaar, RJ; Radivoyevitch, T; Nagata, Y; Khurshed, M; Przychodzen, B; Makishima, H; et al. *IDH1/2* mutations sensitize acute myeloid leukemia to PARP inhibition and this is reversed by IDH1/2-mutant inhibitors. *Clin. Cancer Res.*, 2018, 24, 1705-1715.

[120] Sulkowski, PL; Corso, CD; Robinson, ND; Scanlon, SE; Purshouse, KR; Bai, H; et al. 2-hydroxyglutarate produced neomorphic IDH mutations suppresses homologous recombination and induces PARP inhibitor sensitivity. *Sci. Transl. Med.*, 2017, 9, eaal2463.

[121] Megías-Vericat, JE; Ballesta-López, O; Barragán, E; Montesinos, P. IDH1-mutated relapsed or refractory AML: current challenges and future prospects. *Blood Lymphat. Cancer.*, 2019, 9, 19-32.

[122] Wang, Y; Wild, AT; Turcan, S; Wu, WH; Sigel, C; Klimstra, DS; et al. Targeting therapeutic vulnerabilities with PARP inhibition and radiation in IDH mutant gliomas and cholangiocarcinomas. *Sci. Adv.*, 2020, 6, eaaz3221.

[123] Fritz, C; Portwood, SM; Przespolewski, A; Wang, ES. PARP goes the weasel! Emerging role of PARP inhibitors in acute leukemias. *Blood Rev.*, 2021, 45, 100696.

[124] Platten, M; Bunse, L; Wick, A; Bunse, T; Le Cornet, L; Harting, I; et al. A vaccine targeting mutant IDH1 in newly diagnosed glioma. *Nature.*, 2021, 592, 463-468.

[125] Reardon, DA; Weller, M. Vaccination for IDH-mutant tumors: A novel therapeutic approach applied to glioma. *Med.*, 2021, 2, 450-452.

[126] Schumacher, T; Bunse, L; Pusch, S; Sahm, F; Wiestler, B; Quandt, J; et al. A vaccine targeting mutant IDH1 induces antitumour immunity. *Nature.*, 2014, 512, 324-327.

[127] Duchmann, M; Micol, JB; Duployez, N; Raffoux, E; Thomas, X; Marolleau, JP; et al. Prognostic significance of concurrent gene mutations in intensively treated patients with *IDH* – mutated AML: an ALFA study. *Blood.*, 2021, 137, 2827-2837.

In: New Research on Hematological ...
Editor: David K. Gioia

ISBN: 978-1-53619-955-0
© 2021 Nova Science Publishers, Inc.

Chapter 3

INHIBITION OF NUCLEAR EXPORT AS A NEW THERAPY IN HEMATOLOGIC MALIGNANCIES

Ota Fuchs[*]
Institute of Hematology and Blood Transfusion,
Prague, Czech Republic

ABSTRACT

A nuclear-cytoplasmic transport plays an important role in the development of cancer and drug resistance. Exportin 1 (XPO1) is the major mammalian nuclear export receptor protein, also known as chromosome maintenance 1 (CRM1). XPO1 interacts with Ras-related nuclear protein and with nucleoporins in the nuclear pore complex and transports multiple tumor suppressor proteins (eg p53, FOXO, p21 pRB, BRCA1/2), growth regulators, and oncoprotein mRNAs (eg c-myc, Bcl-xL, MDM2, cyclins) containing a leucine-rich nuclear export signal (NES). XPO1 is also involved in the regulation of cytoplasmic localization and translation of c-myc and other oncoprotein mRNAs (eg cyclin D1, Bcl-6, Mdm2, and Pim) through complexing with eukaryotic initiation factor 4E (eIF4E). The XPO1 protein level is increased in many types of

---

[*] Corresponding Author's E-mail: Ota.Fuchs@uhkt.cz.

cancer including hematological malignancies (multiple myeloma. diffuse large B-cell lymphoma, chronic lymphocytic leukemia, mantle cell lymphoma, T-cell lymphoma, myelodysplastic syndrome, and acute myeloid leukemia). As a result of the increased nuclear-cytoplasmic transport in cancer cells, an elevated level of multiple tumor suppressor proteins and oncoproteins in the cytoplasm leads to advanced disease, resistance to therapy, and poor survival. Thus, XPO1 is a promising cancer drug target. Selinexor (XPOVIO) is the first member of small molecule oral inhibitors of exportin 1 developed for the treatment of cancer. Eltanexor, also known as KPT-8602 or ATG-016, is a member of the second generation of these inhibitors and its anti-leukemic activity was successfully demonstrated in pre-clinical models of acute myeloid leukemia and acute lymphoblastic leukemia. Eltanexor is presently studied in clinical trials in patients with relapsed or refractory multiple myeloma (RRMM) and with intermediate and higher risk myelodysplastic syndrome. Selinexor in combination with synthetic glucocorticoid dexamethasone was approved by the United States Food and Drug Administration (USFDA) on July 3, 2019, for the treatment of adult patients with RRMM who have received at least four prior therapies. Selinexor in combination with bortezomib and dexamethasone was approved in December 2020 for the treatment of adult patients with multiple myeloma who have received at least one prior therapy. Selinexor was also approved by USFDA for the treatment of adult patients with relapsed or refractory diffuse large B-cell lymphoma after at least two lines of systemic therapy. Selinexor is also studied in clinical trials in other hematologic malignancies.

Keywords: nuclear export, nuclear export inhibitors, hematologic malignancies, exportin 1, selinexor, eltanexor

INTRODUCTION

The export of proteins from the nucleus to the cytoplasm plays an important role in the development of cancer and drug resistance [1-3]. The major mammalian nuclear export receptor protein is exportin 1 (XPO1, also known as chromosomal maintenance 1 /CRM1/) [1-5]. The crystal structure of this protein showed a complex with the Ran protein (Ras-related nuclear protein) bound to GTP [6, 7]. XPO1 interacts also with nucleoporins in the nuclear pore complex and transports multiple tumor suppressor proteins (eg p53, FOXO, p21 pRB, BRCA1/2), growth regulators, and oncoprotein mRNAs (eg c-myc, Bcl-xL, MDM2, cyclins) containing a leucine-rich nuclear export signal (NES) (Figure 1) [8]. XPO1 is also involved in the regulation of cytoplasmic localization and translation of c-myc and other oncoprotein mRNAs (eg cyclin D1, Bcl-6, Mdm2, and Pim) through complexing with eukaryotic initiation factor 4E (eIF4E) [9]. The XPO1 protein level is increased in many types of cancer including multiple myeloma [10-13]. As a result of the increased nuclear-cytoplasmic transport in cancer cells, an elevated level of multiple tumor suppressor proteins and oncoproteins in the cytoplasm leads to advanced disease, resistance to therapy, and poor survival. Thus, XPO1 is a promising cancer drug target. Leptomycin B (LMB) is a Streptomyces metabolite that inhibits the function of XPO1 in NES-dependent nuclear export of proteins [14]. However, clinical studies found serious side effects of LMB.

To find a more specific inhibitor of XPO1 without side effects, many natural and synthetic compounds have been tested. These compounds include selinexor (KPT-330, XPOVIO™), verdinexor (KPT-335), KPT-185, KPT-276, KPT-251, and eltanexor (KPT-8602, ATG-016) [15-18]. These agents are a family of small molecules that block nuclear export through covalent binding to cysteine 528 (Cys528) in the cargo proteins NES-binding pocket of exportin1 and contribute to cancer cell death [15]. All these drugs have been developed by Karyopharm Therapeutics Inc., Natick, MA. Verdinexor had anti-tumor activity in dogs with non-Hodgkin lymphoma [19]. Eltanexor was highly active against acute myeloid leukemia (AML) and acute lymphoblastic leukemia (ALL) in vitro and mouse xenograft models [20, 21]. This inhibitor had approximately 30-fold decreased blood-brain barrier penetration in comparison with selinexor in toxicology studies in rats and monkeys. Therefore, eltanexor had a better tolerability profile with reduced the most common adverse events as anorexia, weight loss, and a general feeling of discomfort (a lack of well-being). Eltanexor is presently in clinical trial NCT02649790 in patients with RRMM or higher-risk myelodysplastic syndrome (MDS). Eltanexor under the name ATG-016 is also studied in a clinical trial in patients with intermediate and higher-risk MDS in China.

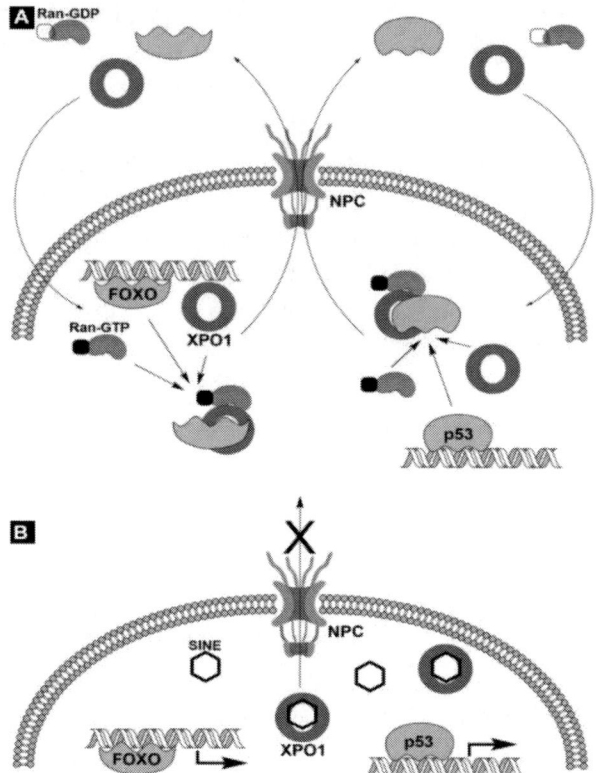

Figure 1. Exportin 1-mediated nuclear export in multiple myeloma; Abbreviations: Ran-GDP and Ran-GTP – GDP or GTP bound Ras related factor; NPC – nuclear pore complex; SINE - selective inhibitor of nuclear export; FOXO – a subgroup of the Forkhead family of transcription factors, p53 – a tumor suppressor protein and transcription factor; XPO1 – exportin 1, also known as chromosomal maintenance 1 (CRM1); (A) XPO1 transports nuclear proteins out of the nucleus. Cargo proteins such as FOXO or p53 that are marked for export from the nucleus bind a pocket in XPO1 in the presence of the activated small G-protein, Ran. The active Ran-GTP-XPO1-cargo complex is exported from the nucleus through the nuclear pore complex driven by the concentration gradient of Ran-GTP across the nuclear membrane. Once in the cytoplasm, Ran-GTP is hydrolyzed to Ran-GDP, and the XPO1-cargo complex dissociates. (B) SINE compounds (Hexagons) bind to XPO1-Cys^{528} and occupy the cargo-binding pocket of XPO1 and prevent formation of the Ran-GTP-XPO1-cargo complex. The result is increased nuclear localization of tumor suppressor cargo proteins and upregulation of their transcriptional activity [15].

SELINEXOR (XPOVIO) FOR THE TREATMENT OF ADULT PATIENTS WITH RELAPSED OR REFRACTORY MULTIPLE MYELOMA

Selinexor is the first member of small-molecule oral inhibitors of exportin 1 developed for the treatment of cancer. The structural formula of selinexor is shown in Figure 2. Selinexor in combination with synthetic glucocorticoid dexamethasone was approved by the FDA (U.S. Food and Drug Administration) on July 3, 2019, for the treatment of adult patients with relapsed or refractory multiple myeloma (RRMM) who have received at least four prior therapies. Selinexor synergizes with dexamethasone and inhibits the mTOR pathway and subsequently induces cell death in multiple myeloma cells [22]. Selinexor increases the expression of glucocorticoid receptor and in combination with dexamethasone stimulates transcriptional activity of the glucocorticoid receptor [22]. Selinexor is studied in clinical trials also in many hematological and solid cancers [23-27]. The treatment with selinexor in preclinical and clinical studies resulted in nuclear localization of tumor suppressor proteins (eg p53 and FOXO3A), induced apoptosis, and decreased proliferation. Selinexor reduces the expression of DNA damage repair proteins and sensitizes cancer cells to DNA damaging agents [28]. Selinexor blocks the transcription factor NF-κB and induces ribosomal stress by disruption of ribosomal subunits assembly [29].

Selinexor is orally bioavailable with a mean half-life of 6-8 h after a single dose. Selinexor pharmacokinetics are not significantly affected by age, sex, ethnicity, renal impairment, or mild hepatic impairment. Most frequent adverse events associated with selinexor treatment are thrombocytopenia, fatigue, nausea, anemia, decreased appetite, anorexia, decreased weight, diarrhea, vomiting, hyponatremia, neutropenia, leukopenia, gastrointestinal toxicity, constipation, dyspnoea, and upper respiratory tract infection. Selinexor can cause fetal harm and should not be administered to a pregnant woman.

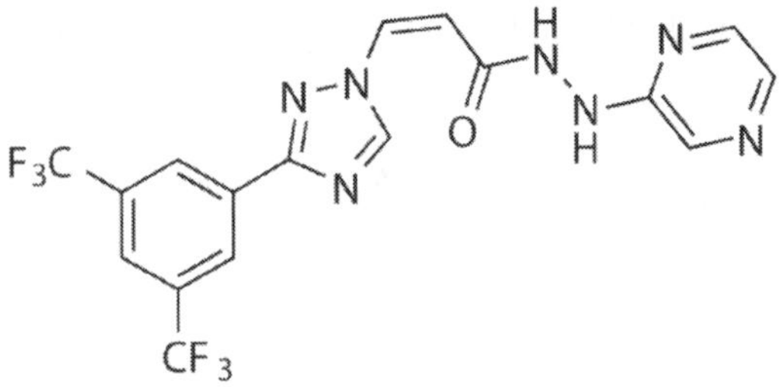

Figure 2. Chemical structure of selinexor (alternative names: ATG-010, KPT-330, ONO7705, XPOVIO, CRM1 nuclear export inhibitor). Chemical name: (Z)-3-(3-(3,5-bis(trifluoromethyl)phenyl-1H-1,2,4-triazol-1-yl)-N´-(pyrazin-2-yl)acrylohydrazide.

THE PHASE II STORM TRIAL WITH SELINEXOR PLUS LOW-DOSE DEXAMETHASONE IN PATIENTS WITH MULTIPLE MYELOMA PRETREATED WITH BORTEZOMIB, CARFILZOMIB, LENALIDOMIDE, POMALIDOMIDE, DARATUMUMAB, AND AN ALKYLATING AGENT

Selinexor demonstrated small single-agent activity with an overall response rate achieved in 4% (2/57 heavily pre-treated patients with RRMM (about six prior therapies) (Table 1) [30]. The response was considerably increased from 4 to 50% (6/12) when selinexor was combined with dexamethasone in a phase I trial in patients with advanced hematological malignancies (NCT 01607892) [30]. The phase II STORM trial (NCT02336815) with selinexor and dexamethasone combination in heavily pre-treated patients with RRMM had relatively quick responses. The primary endpoint was the overall response. Patients were given twice weekly oral doses of selinexor (80 mg) and dexamethasone (20 mg) in 28-day cycles (Table 1) [31, 32]. The overall response was recorded in 21% of patients (16/78) or 26% (32/122) and the median duration of response was 5 months. Patients required a lot of supportive care to manage many side effects. The most common adverse event was thrombocytopenia.

A MULTICENTER, OPEN-LABEL, PHASE 1B/2, DOSE ESCALATION TRIAL STOMP IN PATIENTS WITH RELAPSED OR REFRACTORY MULTIPLE MYELOMA WITH MEDIAN OF THREE PRIOR THERAPIES

The STOMP trial (NCT02343042) is five arms study of selinexor, dexamethasone and either lenalidomide, pomalidomide, bortezomib, carfilzomib, or daratumumab for the treatment of relapsed or refractory multiple myeloma with a median of three prior therapies to evaluate the safety, tolerability, and efficacy of these combinations, determining the maximum tolerated dose, the recommended phase 2 dose, overall response rate (ORR), and progression-free survival (PFS) [26, 27, 29]. Individual arms were described in abstracts No. 726, 1366, and 1393 at ASH 2020 meeting.

THE RANDOMIZED OPEN-LABEL, PHASE III INTERNATIONAL BOSTON TRIAL IN PATIENTS WITH RELAPSED OR REFRACTORY MULTIPLE MYELOMA WITH MEDIAN OF TWO PRIOR THERAPIES

The combination of selinexor and bortezomib once per week plus dexamethasone twice per week (SVd) was compared with bortezomib twice per week in combination with dexamethasone four times per week for the first six months and one half of this dose thereafter (Table 1) [33-35]. The BOSTON study randomly assigned 402 patients with 1 to 3 prior therapies. SVd combination included 195 patients and Vd combination 207 patients. The overall response rate was higher in SVd than Vd (76.4% vs. 62.3%). The primary endpoint was PFS. Median PFS was longer with selinexor treatment: 13.93 months versus 9.46 months in the Vd group. The improvements in survival and response rates with selinexor were associated with higher rates of adverse events (35.9% vs. 17.2% thrombocytopenia; 13.3% vs. 1.0% fatigue; 7.7% vs. 0% nausea) [33-35]. Improvement of PFS was detected in all subgroups, including those with high-risk cytogenetics and those with 17p deletion, where *TP53* could be found.

SELINEXOR PLUS CARFILZOMIB AND DEXAMETHASONE FOR THE TREATMENT OF RELAPSED OR REFRACTORY MULTIPLE MYELOMA

A combination of carfilzomib with dexamethasone was approved for the treatment of patients with RRMM [36, 37]. The clinical benefit rate of the study using a combination of selinexor with carfilzomib and dexamethasone (SKd) was 67% in the first cycle (Table 1) [38]. This study showed the safety and tolerability of the SKd combination twice-weekly. The thrombocytopenia is the main adverse event because selinexor is known to inhibit megakaryocyte maturation [39]. Response rates and time to response were promising in this study. However, the duration of response and progression free survival were shorter than in other selinexor studies. Therapy could take advantage of this combination to overcome resistance, restore disease control and prepare for subsequent therapy.

SELINEXOR IN THERAPY OF PATIENTS WITH RELAPSED OR REFRACTORY CHRONIC LYMPHOCYTIC LEUKEMIA

Selinexor inhibited phosphorylation of several BCR kinases, B cell receptor (BCR) signaling, and signals from the chemokine CXCL12 and its receptor CXCR4 in chronic lymphocytic leukemia (CLL) cells [40]. CLL pathogenesis is based on the prolonged survival and/or resistance to apoptosis of leukemic B cells *in vivo*. The chemokine CXCL12 is normally associated with cell migration. CXCL12 and its receptor CXCR4 stimulate the survival of CLL cells. The tumor suppressor Programmed cell death factor 4 (PDCD4) is one of the phosphorylation targets of CXCL12 signaling [41]. Selinexor showed activity in monotherapy or in combination with ibrutinib [42]. Ibrutinib inhibits Bruton kinase (BTK) in CLL and non-Hodgkin lymphoma. A phase 1 study was accomplished in sixteen relapsed or refractory CLL with a median of four prior therapies (1-14 therapies) [43]. The median age was 60 years (50-80). Together with 16 CLL patients, 8 patients with Richter´s transformation and 6 patients with diffuse large B-cell lymphoma (DLBCL), and 3 patients with mantle cell lymphoma (CML) were studied [43]. Overall 58% of patients received ibrutinib. There were 5 deaths in the course of this study. Three deaths were related to disease progression and two deaths were related to infection. All CLL patients who received prior ibrutinib or had complex karyotype achieved at least stable disease. All patients who did not receive prior ibrutinib had complete remission or partial remission. Two CLL patients with detected BTK mutation had response therapy and seven patients had stable disease. One CLL patient who received 1 prior therapy achieved complete remission with no detectable residual disease.

Walker et al. [44] retrospectively analyzed 1286 CLL cases and found 72 mutations in XPO1 (predominantly E571K and E571G). They created a mouse model with the increased expression of wild-type or mutant XPO1 in B cell compartment. The activity of selinexor will not probably be affected by these mutations because crystal structures of E571 or E571K XPO1 are very similar.

SELINEXOR IN THERAPY OF PATIENTS WITH NON-HODGKIN LYMPHOMA

Non-Hodgkin lymphoma (NHL) subtypes include diffuse large B-cell lymphoma (DLBCL), follicular lymphoma, Richter´s transformation, mantle cell lymphoma, and peripheral T-cell lymphoma. A phase 1 study included 79 patients, 54 patients with DLBCL, and 25 patients with other NHL subtypes, all patients with two or more prior treatments. Four patients with DLBCL, out of 41 evaluated patients, achieved complete remission. Six patients with an extremely aggressive subgroup of DLBCL (approximately 10% of DLBCL) with *MYC, BCL2,* and *BCL6* rearrangements, so-called double or triple hit lymphomas, were also included. Three of these six patients responded to selinexor, one with complete remission, durable at least 35 months [45].

Simultaneous inhibition of exportin 1 and BCL2 is an effective treatment strategy and targeted therapy for double-hit lymphoma including DLBCL [46, 47]. Venetoclax (ABT-199), a potent and selective inhibitor of BCL2 had a very good response in many hematologic malignancies [48-53].

The multicenter, open-label phase 2 SADAL trial evaluated twice-weekly 60-mg selinexor monotherapy administered in 28-day cycles in patients with relapsed or refractory DLBCL, or de novo or transformed follicular lymphoma, after two or more prior therapies (Table 1) [54-56]. A total of 134 patients were enrolled. The objective response rate was the primary endpoint and a value of 29% was obtained. Secondary endpoints were overall survival, duration of response, and safety. A complete remission rate of 13.3% and a partial response rate of 15.7% were found. A total of 8.2% of patients had stable disease and 62.7% had either progressive disease or were not evaluable. The median duration of response was 9.3 months. The median time to at least a partial response was 8.1 weeks. The median overall survival was higher in the younger than 65 years patient group (13.7 months) in comparison with the older than 65 years patient group (7.8 months). The study found that selinexor is also effective in de novo DLBCL and transformed lymphoma (related objective response rates 26.2% and 38.7%). Older patients had lower rates of thrombocytopenia and anemia, but had higher rates of asthenia, nausea, vomiting, and decreased weight than younger patients.

Selinexor in combination with R-CHOP (rituximab, cyclophosphamide, doxorubicin, vincristine, and prednisone) was studied in a phase I trial (NCT03147885) for the treatment of newly diagnosed patients with non-Hodgkin lymphoma (Table 1) [57]. Patients received 6 cycles of R-CHOP with weekly selinexor (60, 80, and 100 mg), then selinexor maintenance treatment for about one year. The median follow-up was 476 days. Analysis of blood samples of enrolled patients detected a decrease of XPO1 and several prosurvival factor levels. The recommended phase II dose was 60 mg selinexor weekly. The most common adverse events were fatigue (67%) and nausea (100%).

T-cell lymphoma (TCL) is a heterogenous subgroup of NHL. Phase 1 study of selinexor in combination with dexamethasone, alkylating agent ifosfamide, carboplatin, and topoisomerase II inhibitor etoposide chemotherapy was done in patients with relapsed or refractory peripheral T-cell or natural-killer/T-cell lymphoma [58]. The combination showed promising complete remission rates but was poorly tolerated. Eleven patients with a median age of 60 years were enrolled. Patients had a median of two prior therapies and seven had primary refractory disease. Grade 3/4 toxicities included thrombocytopenia (82%), anemia (82%), neutropenia (73%, and hyponatremia (73%). Of the ten evaluable patients, nine responded with a complete response and one with a partial response.

SELINEXOR IN MYELOID MALIGNANCIES – ACUTE MYELOID LEUKEMIA AND MYELODYSPLASTIC SYNDROME

The preclinical studies showed that inhibition of XPO1 by selinexor induced apoptosis in acute myeloid leukemia (AML) cells in all phases of the cell cycle [59-62]. Selinexor was then tested in patient-derived xenografts, or PDX models, which are the most sensitive predictors of clinical responses in AML patients [63]. The xenografts were established from AML blasts of patients with a poor prognosis. Selinexor was efficient against leukemia-initiating cells, engrafted into immunodeficient mice and had little cytotoxicity against the normal stem and progenitor cells [64].

Garzon et al. [65] described the phase I trial NCT01607892 with selinexor monotherapy in 95 enrolled patients with relapsed and/or refractory AML (Table 1). The dose of selinexor was increased from 3 to 70 mg/m^2 and was administrated twice weekly as part of a 28-day cycle. The overall response rate was 14% in 81 evaluable patients. The median of the progression-free survival was 1.7 months and the median of the overall survival was 2.7 months. These values were higher in responders (5.1 months and 9.7 months). Thrombocytopenia (19%), anemia (15%), fatigue (14%), and neutropenia (13%) were the most common adverse events possibly related to selinexor. Two patients died in the course of selinexor therapy. Selinexor induced p53 and decreased oncogenic fms-like tyrosine kinase (FLT3) and a cell surface receptor tyrosine kinase KIT.

AML has a wide molecular complexity and therefore it should be treated by a combination of drugs rather than by monotherapy. A phase I study (NCT02573363) of selinexor in combination with high dose cytarabine and mitoxantrone (HiDAC/Mito) enrolled 20 AML patients (12 patients with newly diagnosed and 8 with relapsed/refractory AML; Table 1) [66]. Three (15%) patients received the initial dose of 60 mg of selinexor (about 35 mg/m^2) and 17 (85%) received the target level of 80 mg of selinexor (about 50 mg/m^2). Ten (50%) patients achieved complete remission, 3 patients (15%) achieved complete remission with incomplete recovery, 1 patient (5%) achieved partial remission, and 6 patients (30%) had progressive disease. The recommended phase II dose was 80 mg and justified further study. The increased levels of Wilms tumor 1 (WT1) correlated with bad response or relapse rapidly after induction. No dose-limiting toxicities were observed. Common adverse events encompassed febrile neutropenia (70%), diarrhea (40%), anorexia (30%), electrolyte abnormalities (30%), bacteremia (25%), cardiac toxicities (25%), fatigue (25%), and nausea or vomiting (25%).

Selinexor in combination with decitabine in patients with acute myeloid leukemia was studied in phase I dose-escalation study (NCT02093403) [67]. Twenty-five adult patients with relapsed or refractory AML and older untreated patients (age at least 60 years) with AML were treated with a dose of 60 mg selinexor weekly for two weeks after decitabine (20 mg/m^2). The overall response was 40% and the most common grade (3 and higher) toxicities were asymptomatic hyponatremia (68%), febrile neutropenia (44%), sepsis (44%), hypophosphatemia (36%), and pneumonia (28%).

Combinatorial targeting of XPO1 and FLT3 had synergistic anti-leukemia effects through induction of differentiation and apoptosis in *FLT3*-mutated AML [68]. The combination of selinexor and sorafenib induced anti-leukemia efficacy in a human *FLT3*-mutated xenograft model. A phase IB clinical trial with this combination in 14 patients with refractory AML induced complete/partial remissions in six of 14 AML patients, who received a median of three prior therapies (NCT02530476). This study showed marked pro-apoptotic effects of selinexor in combination with sorafenib against AML with *FLT3*-ITD and/or TKD mutations (Table 1). Selinexor was also studied in combination with other inhibitors of *FLT3*-mutated AML (midostaurin and gilteritinib) [69].

The efficacy of BCL-2 inhibitor venetoclax in AML was mentioned [49, 52]. The combination of selinexor and venetoclax synergistically induced apoptosis in AML cell lines and primary AML patient samples [70]. Selinexor decreased the level of anti-apoptotic protein Mcl-1 of the BCL-2 family and increased the binding of Mcl-1 to Bim. This second effect of selinexor of preventing Bim from inducing apoptosis was overcome by venetoclax. The combination of selinexor and venetoclax overcome in this way apoptosis resistance of AML cells.

A randomized, open-label, phase 2 study of selinexor versus physician´s choice (PC) in relapsed/refractory AML patients (SOPRA-Selinexor in Older (60 years and older; Table 1) Patients with Relapsed/Refractory AML; NCT02088541) was carried out. Of the 317 randomized patients, 297 patients received at least 1 dose of study drug-selinexor (60 mg twice per week) or best supportive care (BSC) alone, or BSC plus either azacitidine or decitabine, or low dose cytosine arabinoside, and were included in the safety population. The primary endpoint of this study was the overall survival of selinexor therapy compared to PC. The target was a 75% improvement in overall survival from 3.0 months in the PC arm to 5.2 months in the selinexor arm. The primary endpoint was not achieved. There was no significant difference in median overall survival in selinexor arm in comparison with the PC arm. There were 11.9% complete remission or complete remission with incomplete recovery in patients treated with selinexor versus 3.5% on PC. AML patients on selinexor who achieved complete remission or complete remission with incomplete recovery had improved survival (median 397 days) compared to all rest enrolled AML patients. The most common treatment-emergent adverse events in the selinexor arm were nausea, anorexia, fatigue, diarrhea, thrombocytopenia, vomiting, and pyrexia.

Patients with high-risk MDS resistant to azacitidine or decitabine have very short overall survival (less than 6 months). Preclinical studies showed that inhibition of exportin 1 blocked NF-κB signaling and stimulated p53 accumulation. Both these effects induced apoptosis of

MDS cells. A phase 2 trial studied the safety and activity of selinexor in patients with MDS or oligoblastic AML refractory to hypomethylating agents [71, 72]. It was a single-center (the Memorial Sloan Kettering Cancer Center, New York), single-arm study registered with Clinical Trials.gov. NCT02228525. Twenty-five patients with 20-30% blasts and refractory to hypomethylating agents received oral selinexor in cycles (60 mg twice per week for 2 weeks followed by 1 week without selinexor as one cycle). The median follow-up was 8.5 months. Six patients from the 23 evaluable patients had complete remission in the bone marrow and 12 patients achieved stable disease. Thrombocytopenia (32%) and hyponatremia (20%) were the most common grade 3 or 4 adverse events.

CONCLUSION AND PERSPECTIVES

Encouraging results with selinexor and other selective inhibitors of nuclear export will likely be more effective in combination with various agents, including ibrutinib, immune-checkpoint inhibitors, mTOR inhibitors, gemcitabine, or anthracyclines. Numerous trials are currently planned, organized or ongoing to test synergistic effects in patients with drug-resistant cancers [17, 73, 74]. The inhibition of exportin1 affects the 3D nuclear organization of telomeres in tumor cells, while normal cells are minimally affected [75]. Therefore, the 3D nuclear organization of telomeres is a sensitive indicator of cellular response when treated with selinexor, eltanexor, and other selective inhibitors of nuclear export. The most commonly reported toxicities were low-grade gastrointestinal adverse events, which are dose- limiting. Unusual toxicities such as hyponatremia and blurred vision may be a class-effect phenomenon. Frequent monitoring of serum electrolytes of all patients treated with selective inhibitors of nuclear export is needed. High-throughput screening of potential combination therapies together with CRISPR-based, genome-wide library screening is necessary [76-79].

Table 1. Clinical trials with selective inhibitors of nuclear export in hematological malignancies

Chemotherapy	Disease	Phase	Reference
Treatment with selinexor and low dose bortezomib plus dexamethasone	*RRMM (quad and penta refractory)*	1/2	29
Treatment with selinexor and dexamethasone	RRMM (about six prior therapies) and Waldenstrom macroglobulinemia	2 (STORM trial)	30-32
Treatment with selinexor, bortezomib, and dexamethasone Treatment with selinexor, carfilzomib, and dexamethasone	RRMM RRMM	3 (BOSTON trial) 1	33-35 38
Treatment with selinexor and ibrutinib Treatment with selinexor Treatment with selinexor	RRCLL agressive non-Hodgkin lymhoma non-Hodgkin lymphoma Diffuse large B-cell lymphoma	Phase 1 (NCT02303392) 1 2 (SADAL trial)	43 45 54-56
Treatment with selinexor and R-CHOP	non-Hodgkin lymphoma	1 (NCT03147885)	57
Treatment with selinexor and dexamethasone, alkylating agent ifosfamide, carboplatin, and topoisomerase II inhibitor etoposide	RRT-cell lymphoma or or natural-killer/T-cell lymphoma	1	
Treatment with selinexor Treatment with selinexor in combination with high dose cytarabine and mitoxantrone (HiDAC/Mito)	RRAML newly diagnosed and RRAML	1 (NCT01607892) 1 (NCT02573363)	65 66
Treatment with selinexor and sorafenib	*FLT3*-mutated RRAML	1 (NCT02530476)	68
Treatment with selinexor versus physician´s choice (PC)	RRAML	2 (SOPRA trial) (NCT02088541)	
Treatment with selinexor	high-risk MDS resistant to azacitidine or decitabine	2 (NCT02228525)	71, 72

Despite encouraging results, the optimism must be mixed with caution. Some unwanted oncogenes are bound to be retained in the nucleus, causing an unfavorable balance between tumor suppressor proteins and oncogenes. High-throughput proteomic approaches may help to evaluate results and consequences of this nuclear retention of proteins associated with selective inhibitors of nuclear export therapy.

ACKNOWLEDGMENTS

This work was supported by the project for conceptual development of research organization No 00023736 (Institute of Hematology and Blood Transfusion) from the Ministry of Health of the Czech Republic.

REFERENCES

[1] Turner JG, Sullivan DM. CRM1 mediated nuclear export of proteins and drug resistance in cancer. *Curr. Med. Chem.* 2008; 15: 2648-2655.

[2] Nguen KT, Holloway MP, Altura RA. The CRM1 nuclear export protein in normal development and disease. *Int. J. Biochem. Mol. Biol.* 2012; 3: 137-151.

[3] Turner JG, Dawson J, Cubitt CL, Baz R, Sullivan DM. Inhibition of CRM1-dependent nuclear export sensitizes malignant cells to cytotoxic and targeted agents. *Semin. Cancer Biol.* 2014; 27: 62-73.

[4] Gravina GL, Senapedis W, Mc Cauley D, Baloglu E, Shacham S, Festuccia C. Nucleo-cytoplasmic transport as a therapeutic target of cancer. *J. Hematol. Oncol.* 2014; 7: 85.

[5] Lu C, Figueroa JA, Liu Z, Konala V, Aulakh A, Verma R, et al. Nuclear export as a novel therapeutic target: the CRM1 connection. *Curr. Cancer Drug Targets.* 2015; 15: 575-592.

[6] Monecke T, Güttler T, Neumann P, Dickmanns A, Görlich D, Ficner R. Crystal structure of the nuclear export receptor CRM1 in complex with Snurportin1 and RanGTP. *Science.* 2009; 324: 1087-1091.

[7] Monecke T, Dickmanns A, Ficner R. Allosteric control of the exportin CRM1 unraveled by crystal structure analysis. *FEBS J.* 2014; 281: 4179-4194.

[8] Fung HY, Chook YM. Atomic basis of CRM1-cargo recognition, release and inhibition. *Semin. Cancer Biol.* 2014; 27: 52-61.

[9] Volpon L, Culjkovic-Kraljacic B, Sohn HS, Blanchet-Cohen A, Osborne MJ, Borden KLB. A biochemical framework for eIF4E-dependent mRNA export and nuclear recycling of the export machinery. *RNA.* 2017; 23: 927-937.

[10] Schmidt J, Braggio E, Kortuem KM, Egan JB, Zhu YX, Xin CS, et al. Genome-wide studies in multiple myeloma identify XPO1/CRM1 as a critical target validated using the selective nuclear export inhibitor KPT-276. *Leukemia.* 2013; 27: 2357-2365.

[11] Muqbil I, Azmi AS, Mohammad RM. Nuclear export inhibition for pancreatic cancer therapy. *Cancers* (Basel). 2018; 10: 138.

[12] Chanukuppa V, Paul D, Taunk K, Chatterjee T, Sharma S, Kumar S, et al. XPO1 is a critical player for bortezomib resistance in multiple myeloma: A quantitative proteomic approach. *J. Proteomics.* 2019; 209: 103504.

[13] Taylor J, Sendino M, Gorelick AN, Pastore A, Chang MT, Penson AV, et al. Altered nuclear export signal recognition as a driver of oncogenesis. *Cancer Disc.* 2019; 9: 1452-1467.

[14] Kudo N, Wolff B, Sekimoto T, Schreiner EP, Yoneda Y, Yanagida M, et al. Leptomycin B inhibition of signal-mediated nuclear export by direct binding to CRM1. *Exp. Cell Res.* 1998; 242: 540-547.

[15] Parikh K, Cang S, Sekhri A, Liu D. Selective inhibitors of nuclear export (SINE)-a novel class of anti-cancer agents. *J. Hematol. Oncol.* 2014; 7: 78.

[16] Gandhi UH, Senapedis W, Baloglu E, Unger TJ, Chari A, Vogl D, Cornell RF. Clinical implications of targeting XPO1-mediated nuclear export in multiple myeloma. *Clin. Lymphoma Myeloma Leuk.* 2018; 18: 335-345.

[17] Allegra A, Innao V, Allegra AG, Leanza R, Musolino C. Selective inhibitors of nuclear export in the treatment of hematologic malignancies. *Clin. Lymphoma Myeloma Leuk.* 2019; 19: 689-698.

[18] Nachmias B, Schimmer AD. Targeting nuclear import and export in hematological malignancies. *Leukemia.* 2020; 34: 2875-2886.

[19] Sadowski AR, Gardner HL, Borgatti A, Wilson H, Vail DM, Lachowicz J, et al. Phase II study of the oral selective selective inhibitor of nuclear export (SINE) KPT-335 (verdinexor) in dogs with lymphoma. *BMC Vet. Res.* 2018; 14: 250.

[20] Etchin J, Berezovskaya A, Conway AS, Galinsky JA, Stone RM, Baloglu E, et al. KPT-8602, a second-generation inhibitor of XPO1-mediated nuclearexport, is well tolerated and highly active against AML blasts and leukemia-initiating cells. *Leukemia.* 2017; 31: 143-150.

[21] Vercruysse T, De Bie J, Neggers JE, Jacquemyn M, Vanstreels E, Schmid-Burgk JL, et al. The second-generation exportin-1 inhibitor KPT-8602 demonstrates potent activity against acute lymphoblastic leukemia. *Clin. Cancer Res.* 2017; 23:2528-2541.

[22] Argueta C, Kashyap T, Klebanov B, Unger TJ, Guo C, Harrington S, et al. Selinexor synergizes with dexamethasone to repress mTORC1 signaling and induce multiple myeloma cell death. *Oncotarget.* 2018; 9: 25529-25544.

[23] Syed YY. Selinexor: first global approval. *Drugs.* 2019; 79: 1485-1494.

[24] Peterson TJ, Orozco J, Buege M. Selinexor: A first-in-class nuclear export inhibitor for management of multiply relapsed multiple myeloma. *Ann. Pharmacother.* 2020; 54: 577-582.

[25] Podar K, Shah J, Chari A, Richardson PG, Jagannath S. Selinexor for the treatment of multiple myeloma. *Expert Opin. Pharmacother.* 2020; 21: 398-408.

[26] Richter J, Madduri D, Richard S, Chari A. Selinexor in relapsed/refractory multiple myeloma. *Ther. Adv. Hematol.* 2020; 11: 1-10.

[27] Benkova K, Mihalyova J, Hajek R, Jelinek T. Selinexor, selective inhibitor of nuclear export: unselective bullet for blood cancers. *Blood Rev.* 2021; 46: 100758.

[28] Kashyap T, Argueta C, Unger TJ, Klebanov B, Debler S, Senapedis W, et al. Selinexor reduces the expression of DNA damage repair proteins and sensitizes cancer cells to DNA damaging agents. *Oncotarget.* 2018; 9: 30773-30786.

[29] Bahlis NJ, Sutherland H, White D, Sebag M, Lentzsch S, Kotb R, et al. Selinexor plus low-dose bortezomib and dexamethasone for patients with relapsed or refractory multiple myeloma. *Blood*. 2018; 132: 2546-2554.

[30] Chen C, Siegel D, Guttierrez M, Jacoby M, Hofmeister CC, Gabrail N, et al. Safety and efficacy of selinexor in relapsed or refractory multiple myeloma and Waldenstrom macroglobulinemia. *Blood*. 2018; 131: 855-863.

[31] Vogl DT, Dingli D, Cornell RF, Huff CA, Jagannath S, Bhutani D, et al. Selective inhibition of nuclear export with oral selinexor for treatment of relapsed or refractory multiple myeloma. *J. Clin. Oncol*. 2018; 36: 859-866.

[32] Chari A, Vogl DT, Gavriatopoulou M, Naoka AK, Yee AJ, Huff CA, et al. Oral selinexor-dexamethasone for triple class refractory multiple myeloma. *N. Engl. J. Med*. 2019; 381: 727-738.

[33] Grosicki S, Simonova M, Spicka I, Pour L, Kriachok I, Gavriatopoulou M, et al. Once-per-week selinexor, bortezomib, and dexamethasone versus twice-per-week bortezomib dexamethasone in patients with multiple myeloma (BOSTON): a randomised, open-label, phase 3 trial. *Lancet*. 2020; 396: 1563-1573.

[34] Mateos MV, Gavriatopoulou M, Facon T, Auner HW, Leleu X, Hájek R, et al. Effect of prior treatments on selinexor, bortezomib, and dexamethasone in previously treated multiple myeloma. *J. Hematol. Oncol*. 2021; 14: 59.

[35] Auner HW, Gavriatopoulou M, Delimpasi S, Simonova M, Spicka I, Pour L, et al. Effect of age and frailty on the efficacy and tolerability of once-weekly selinexor, bortezomib, and dexamethasone in previously treated multiple myeloma. *Am. J. Hematol*. 2021; doi: 10.1002/ajh.26172.

[36] Dimopoulos MA, Moreau P, Palumbo A, Joshua D, Pour L, Hajek R, et al. Carfilzomib and dexamethasone versus bortezomib and dexamethasone for patients with relapsed or refractory multiple myeloma (ENDEAVOR): a randomised, phase 3, open-label, multicentre study. *Lancet Oncol*. 2016; 17: 27-38.

[37] Dimopoulos MA, Goldshmidt H, Niesvizky R, Joshua D, Chng WJ, Oriol A, et al. Carfilzomib or bortezomib in relapsed or refractory

multiple myeloma (ENDEAVOR): an interim overall survival analysis of an open-label, randomised, phase 3 trial. *Lancet Oncol.* 2017; 18: 1327-1337.

[38] Jakubowiak AJ, Jasielec JK, Rosenbaum CA, Cole CE, Chari A, Mikhael J, et al. Phase 1 study of selinexor plus carfilzomib and dexamethasone for the treatment of relapsed/refractory multiple myeloma. *Brit. J. Haematol.* 2019; 186: 549-560.

[39] Machlus KR, Wu SK, Vijey P, Soussou TS, Liu ZJ, Shacham E, et al. Selinexor- induced thrombocytopenia results from inhibition of thrombopoietin signaling in early megakaryopoiesis. *Blood.* 2017; 130: 1132-1143.

[40] Zhong Y, El-Gamal D, Dubovsky JA, Beckwith RA, Harrington BK, Williams KE, et al. Selinexor suppresses downstream effectors of B-cell activation, proliferation and migration in chronic lymphocytic leukemia cells. *Leukemia.* 2014; 28: 1158-1163.

[41] O´Hayre M, Salanga CL, Kipps TJ, Messmer D, Dorrestein PC, Handel TM. Elucidating the CXCl12/CXCR4 signaling network in chronic lymphocytic leukemia through phosphoproteomics analysis. *PLoS One* 2010; 5: e11716.

[42] Hing ZA, Mantel R, Beckwith KA, Guinn D, Williams E, Smith LL, et al. Selinexor is effective in acquired resistance to ibrutinib and synergizes with ibrutinib in chronic lymphocytic leukemia. *Blood.* 2015; 125: 3128-3132.

[43] Stephens DM, Huang Y, Agyeman A, Ruppert AS, Boyu H, Turner N, et al. Selinexor combined with ibrutinib demonstrates tolerability and efficacy in advanced B-cell malignancies: a phase I study. *Blood.* 2019; 134 (Suppl. 1): 4310.

[44] Walker JS, Hing YA, Harrington B, Baumhardt J, Ozer HG, Lehman A, et al. Recurrent XPO1 mutations alter pathogenesis of chronic lymphocytic leukemia. *J. Hematol. Oncol.* 2021; 14: 17.

[45] Kuruvilla J, Savona M, Bay R, Mau-Sorensen PM, Gabrail N, Garzon R, et al. Selective inhibition of nuclear export with selinexor in patients with non-Hodgkin lymphoma. *Blood.* 2017; 129: 3175-3183.

[46] Liu Y, Azizian NG, Dou Y, Pham LV, Li Y. Simultaneous targeting of XPO1 and BCL2 as an effective treatment strategy for double-hit lymphoma. *J. Hematol. Oncol.* 2019; 12: 119.

[47] Fischer MA, Friedlander SY, Arrate MP, Chang H, Gorska AE, Fuller LD, et al. Venetoclax response is enhanced by selective inhibitor of nuclear export compounds in hematologic malignancies. *Blood Adv.* 2020; 4: 586-598.

[48] Souers AJ, Leverson JD, Boghaert ER, Ackler SL, Catron ND, Chen J, et al. ABT-199, a potent and selective BCL-2 inhibitor, achieves antitumor activity while sparing platelets. *Nat. Med.* 2013; 19: 202-208.

[49] Pan R, Hogdal LJ, Benito JM, Bucci D, Han L, Borthakur G, et al. Selective BCL-2 inhibition by ABT-199 causes on-target cell death in acute myeloid leukemia. *Cancer Discov.* 2014; 4: 362-375.

[50] Davids MS, Roberts AW, Seymour JF, Pagel JM, Kahl BS, Wierda WG, et al. Phase 1 first-in-human study of venetoclax in patients with relapsed or refractory non-Hodgkin lymphoma. *J. Clin. Oncol.* 2017; 35: 826-833.

[51] Roberts AW, Davids MS, Pagel JM, Kahl BS, Puvvada SD, Gerecitano JF, et al. Targeting BCL2 with venetoclax in relapsed chronic lymphocytic leukemia. *N. Engl. J. Med.* 2016; 374: 311-322.

[52] Konopleva M, Pollyea DA, Potluri J, Chyla B, Hogdal L, Busman T, et al. Efficacy and biological correlates of response in a phase II study of venetoclax monotherapy in patients with acute myelogenous leukemia. *Cancer Discov.* 2016; 6: 1106-1117.

[53] DiNardo CD, Pratz KW, Letai, A, Jonas BA, Wei AH, Thirman M, et al. Safety and preliminary efficacy of venetoclax wsith decitabine or azacitidine in elderly patients with previously untreated acute myeloid leukaemia: a non-randomised, open-label, phase 1b study. *Lancet Oncol.* 2018; 19: 216-228.

[54] Kalakonda N, Maerevoet M, Cavallo F, Follows G, Goy A, Vermaat JSP, et al. Selinexor in patients with relapsed or refractory diffuse large B-cell lymphoma (SADAL): a single-arm, multinational, multicentre, open-label, phase 2 trial. *Lancet Haematol.* 2020; 7: e511-522.

[55] Maerevoet M, Vermaat JSP, Canales MA, Casasnovas R-O, Van Den Neste E, Goy A, et al. Single agent oral selinexor demonstrates deep and durable responses in relapsed/refractory diffuse large B-cell lymphoma (DLBCL) in both GCB and non-

GCB subtypes: the phase 2b Sadal study. *Blood.* 2018; 132: 1677.

[56] Kalakonda N, Cavallo F, Follows G, Goy A, Vermaat JSP, Casasnovas R-O, et al. A phase 2b study of selinexor in patients with relapsed/refractory (R/R) diffuse large B-cell lymphoma (DLBCL). *Clin. Lymhoma Myeloma Leuk.* 2019; 19: S248-249.

[57] Seymour EK, Khan HY, Li Y, Chaker, M, Muqbil I, Aboukameel A, et al. Selinexor in combination with R-CHOP for frontline treatment of non-Hodgkin lymphoma: results of a phase I study. *Clin. Cancer Res.* 2021; doi: 10.1158/1078-0432.CCR-20-4929.

[58] Tang T, Martin P, Somasundaram N, Lim C, Tao M, Poon E, et al. Phase 1 study of selinexor in combination with dexamethasone, ifosfamide, carboplatin, etoposide chemotherapy in patients with relapsed or refractory peripheral T-cell or natural-killer/T-cell lymphoma. *Haematologica.* 2020; doi: 10.3324/haematol. 2020. 251454.

[59] Ranganathan P, Yu X, Na C, Santhanam R, Shacham S, Kauffman M, et al. Preclinical activity of a novel CRM1 inhibitor in acute myeloid leukemia. *Blood.* 2012; 120: 1765-1773.

[60] Kojima K, Kornblau SM, Ruvolo V, Dilip A, Duvvuri S, Davis RE, et al. Prognostic impact and targeting of CRM1 in acute myeloid leukemia. *Blood.* 2013; 121: 4166-4174.

[61] Etchin J, Sanda T, Mansour MR, Kentis A, Montero J, Le BT, et al. KPT-330 inhibitor of CRM1 (XPO1)-mediated nuclear export has selective anti-leukaemic activity in preclinical models of T-cell acute lymphoblastic lekaemia and acute myeloid leukemia. *Br. J. Haematol.* 2013; 161: 117-127.

[62] Etchin J, Sun Q, Kentis A, Farmer A, Zhang ZC, Sanda T, et al. Antileukemic activity of nuclear export inhibitors that spare normal hematopoietic cells. *Leukemia.* 2013; 27: 66-74.

[63] Sarry JE, Murphy K, Perry R, Sanchez PV, Secreto A, Keefer C, et al. Human acute myelogenous leukemia stem cells are rare and heterogeneous when assayed in NOD/SCID/IL2Rγc-deficient mice. *J. Clin. Invest.* 2011; 121: 384-395.

[64] Etchin J, Montero J, Berezovskaya A, Le BT, Kentis A, Christie AL, et al. Activity of a selective inhibitor of nuclear export,

selinexor (KPT-330), against AML-initiating cells engrafted into immunosuppressed NSG mice. *Leukemia.* 2016; 30: 190-199.

[65] Garzon R, Savona M, Baz R, Andreeff M, Gabrail N, Gutierrez M, et al. A phase I clinical trial of single-agent selinexor in acute myeloid leukemia. *Blood.* 2017; 129: 3165-3174.

[66] Wang AY, Weiner H, Green M, Chang H, Fulton N, Larson RA, et al. A phase I study of selinexor in combination with high dose cytarabine and mitoxantrone for remission induction in patients with acute myeloid leukemia. *J. Hematol. Oncol.* 2018; 11: 4.

[67] Bhatnagar B, Zhao Q, Mims AM, Vasu S, Behbeham GK, Larkin K, et al. Selinexor in combination with decitabine in patients with acute myeloid leukemia results from a phase 1 study. *Leuk. Lymphoma.* 2020; 61: 387-396.

[68] Zhang W, Ly C, Ishizawa J, Mu H, Ruvolo V, Shacham S, et al. Combinatorial targeting of XPO1 and FLT3 exerts synergistic anti-leukemia effects through induction of differentiation and apoptosis in *FLT3*-mutated acute myeloid leukemias: from concept to clinical trial. *Haematologica.* 2018; 103: 1642-1653.

[69] Brinton LT, Sher S, Williams K, Canfield D, Orwick S, Wasmuth R, et al. Cotargeting of XPO1 enhances the antileukemic activity of midostaurin and gilteritinib in acute myeloid leukemia. *Cancers.* 2020; 12: 1574.

[70] Luedtke DA, Su Y, Liu S, Edwards H, Wang Y, Lin H, et al. Inhibition of XPO1 enhances cell death induced by ABT-199 in acute myeloid leukaemia via Mcl-1. *J. Cell. Mol. Med.* 2018; 22: 6099-6111.

[71] Sockel K. Treating myelodysplastic syndromes by nuclear transport inhibition. *Lancet Haematol.* 2020; 7: e552-e553.

[72] Taylor J, Mi X, Penson AV, Paffenholz SC, Alvarez K, Siegler A, et al. Safety and activity of selinexor in patients with myelodysplastic syndromes or oligoblastic acute myeloid leukaemia refractory to hypomethylating agents: a single-centre, single-arm, phase 2 trial. *Lancet Haematol.* 2020; 7: e566-e574.

[73] Azmi AS, Mohammad RM. Targeting cancer at the nuclear pore. *J. Clin. Oncol.* 2016; 34: 4180-4182.

[74] Azmi AS, Mohammed HU, Mohammad RM. The nuclear export protein XPO1-from biology to targeted therapy. *Nature Rev. Clin. Oncol.* 2021; 18: 152-169.

[75] Taylor-Kashton C, Lichtensztejn D, Baloglu E, Senapedis W, Shacham S, Kauffman MG, et al. XPO1 inhibition preferentially disrupts the 3D nuclear organization of telomeres in tumor cells. *J. Cell. Physiol.* 2016; 231: 2711-2719.

[76] Shalem O, Sanjana NE, Hartenian E, Shi X, Scott DA, Mikkelson T, et al. Genome-scale CRISPR-Cas9 knockout screening in human cells. *Science.* 2014; 343: 84-87.

[77] Mathews Griner LA, Guha R, Shinn P, Young RM, Keller JM, Liu D, et al. High-throughput combinatorial screening identifies drugs that cooperate with ibrutinib to kill activated B cell-like diffuse large B-cell lymphoma cells. *Proc. Natl. Acad. Sci. USA.* 2014; 111: 2349-2354.

[78] Doench JG. Am I ready for CRISPR? A user´s guide to genetic screens. *Nat. Rev. Genet.* 2018; 19: 67-80.

[79] Hanna RE, Doench JG. Design and analysis of CRISPR-Cas experiments. *Nat. Biotechnol.* 2020; 38: 813-823.

In: New Research on Hematological ...
Editor: David K. Gioia
ISBN: 978-1-53619-955-0
© 2021 Nova Science Publishers, Inc.

Chapter 4

POLY(ADP-RIBOSE) POLYMERASE INHIBITORS IN THE TREATMENT OF MYELODYSPLASTIC SYNDROME AND ACUTE MYELOID LEUKEMIA

Ota Fuchs[*]

Institute of Hematology and Blood Transfusion,
Prague, Czech Republic

ABSTRACT

The Poly(ADP-ribose) polymerase (PARP) family of 18 proteins has important functions in cellular processes such as the regulation of chromatin remodeling, transcription, apoptosis, stress response, and DNA damage response. PARP-1 is a critical DNA repair enzyme in the base excision repair pathway and an attractive target in cancer therapy. Lynparza (olaparib) and other PARP inhibitors (PARPi) had anti-proliferative and pro-apoptotic effects in human acute myeloid leukemia (AML) blasts at concentrations that do not affect the viability of normal bone marrow stem cells. Although PARPi can generally slow leukemic cell growth, PARPi treatment of RUNX1-RUNXT1, promyelocytic

---

[*] Corresponding Author's E-mail: Ota.Fuchs@uhkt.cz.

leukemia-retinoic acid receptor-α (PML-RARα) fusion genes bearing AML cells resulted in their morphological differentiation into monocytic and granulocytic lineages, which was consistent with leukemic differentiation induced by excessive DNA damage. These chromosomal translocations could weaken the homologous recombination repair activity and sensitize AML cells to PARPi treatment. Olaparib cytotoxicity on primary AML blasts was caused by drug-induced DNA damage, upregulation of death receptors, and transcription factor NF-κB activation. PARP inhibitors induced anti-leukemic effects also in *FLT3-ITD* AML, where PARPi and FLT3 inhibitors showed synergistic effect. *IDH* mutations also sensitize AML cells to PARP inhibitors. PARP contributes to immune evasion of anti-tumor immune cells by PARP-dependent apoptosis through increased reactive oxygen species (ROS) and by PARP-mediated downregulation of natural killer cell-activating receptor-ligand (NKG2DL) expression on AML cells. PARPi reversed the ROS-induced apoptosis of NK and T cells. High-risk myelodysplastic syndrome (MDS) cases are associated with a decrease of apoptosis and high levels of genomic instability caused by alterations in DNA damage response pathways. Olaparib as a single agent or in combination with hypomethylating agents (decitabine or azacitidine) was not only cytotoxic, but also stimulated differentiation of immature MDS myeloid cells. Recently, proteolysis targeting chimera (PROTAC) for PARP-1 degradation was designed.

Keywords: acute myeloid leukemia, myelodysplastic syndrome, poly(ADP-ribose) polymerase, PARP inhibitor, olaparib, DNA-damage, synthetic lethality, PARP1 trapping, DNA-repair

INTRODUCTION

Myelodysplastic syndromes (MDS) are a group of age-associated heterogeneous clonal hematopoietic disorders characterized by ineffective hematopoiesis with peripheral cytopenias, dysplasia in one or more hematopoietic cell lineages, and a differentiation deffect, with an increased risk of progression to AML [1-8]. MDS are associated with genomic instability and extensive DNA damage caused by deficient repair mechanisms [9-20]. Aberrations in DNA damage response/repair genes other than *TP53* and some genes involved in DNA damage checkpoints are rare. Differential expression of homologous recombination DNA repair-associated genes during MDS progression was detected and could be confirmed as new biomarkers related to pathogenesis and poor prognosis in MDS [11, 14-17].

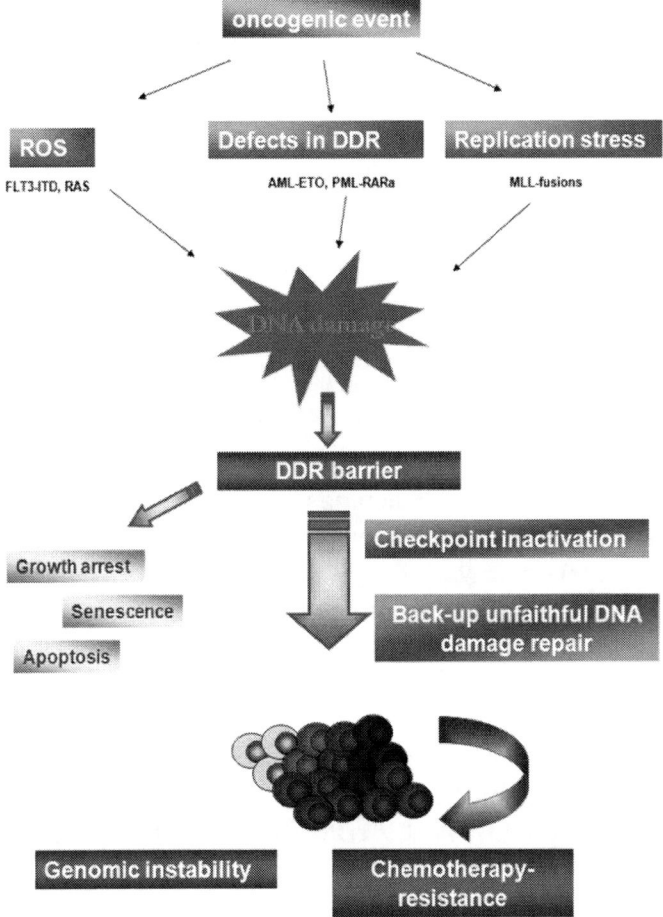

Figure 1. Aberrant DNA damage repair in AML cells. Recurrent chromosomal translocations in AML induce the leukemogenesis through deregulation of DNA damage repair genes. DNA damage is also induced by replicative and oxidative stress and is accumulated in AML cells [22]. Conversely, aberrant DNA damage response might be associated with a chemoresistant phenotype. Abbreviations: DDR-DNA damage response, ROS-reactive oxygen species.

The characteristic feature of cancer is genomic instability and MDS is associated with chromosomal abnormalities and mutations in up to 94% of cases [21]. Increased DNA damage and alteration of the DNA damage response (DDR) are critical features of genetic instability presumably implicated in pathogenesis of MDS and AML. A continuous increase of DNA double-strand breaks (DSB) was found in conjunction with an impaired DDR in MDS and AML [22]. Cytotoxic therapy results in the expansion of clones carrying mutations in DNA damage response genes, including TP53 and PPM1D (protein phosphatase Mn^{2+}/Mg^{2+}-dependent 1D). PPM1D is a DNA damage response regulator that is frequently mutated in clonal hematopoiesis. Mutations in PPM1D were present in 20% of patients with therapy-related AML or MDS [23-25].

The vast majority of *de novo* AML present unaltered *TP53* alleles. However, *TP53* mutations are frequently detected in AML related to increased genomic instability, such as therapy-related (t-AML) or AML with myelodysplasia-related changes. Of note, *TP53* mutations are associated with complex cytogenetic abnormalities, advanced age, chemoresistance, and poor outcomes [26-31]. Epigenetic silencing of DDR genes could contribute to leukemogenesis. In addition, a variety of AML oncogenes have been shown to induce replication and oxidative stress leading to accumulation of DNA damage, which affects the balance between proliferation and differentiation (Figure 1). In opposition to the silencing of DDR genes, their upregulation is associated with escape mechanisms of AML cells to the DDR and induces chemotherapy resistance [32].

The nuclear enzyme poly(ADP-ribose) polymerase 1 (PARP1) and PARP2 play important roles in DNA repair [33, 34]. PARP family contains 18 members, but only PARP1 and PARP2 catalytic activity is immediately induced by DNA strand breaks [35]. PARP inhibitor functions as a competitive inhibitor of nicotinamide adenine dinucleotide (NAD+) at the catalytic site of PARP1 and PARP2 enzymes. These enzymes are induced by single-strand breaks (SSBs) of the damaged DNA and are involved in the base excision repair (BER) pathway. PARP inhibitors mediate their antitumor effects as catalytic inhibitors that block the repair of DNA SSBs. Inhibition of the BER pathway by PARP inhibitor leads to the accumulation of unpaired

SSBs, which leads to the formation of deleterious double-strand breaks (DSBs). In cells with intact homologous recombination repair deficiencies, PARP inhibitor causes synthetic lethality through the combination of two molecular events that are otherwise nonlethal when occurring in isolation (Figure 2) [36, 37].

POLY(ADP-RIBOSE) POLYMERASE SUPERFAMILY

The poly(ADP-ribose) (PAR) polymerases (PARPs) are a superfamily of enzymes that share the ability to catalyze the transfer of ADP-ribose to target proteins/poly(ADP-ribosyl)ation/. The members of the PARP family are encoded by different genes, and share homology in a conserved catalytic domain. Although some isoforms including PARP1 and PARP2 are best known for their involvement in DNA repair processes [38-44], it is now clear that these and other PARPs have an important role in several cellular processes including cell proliferation and cell death [45-50]. Many cellular substrates for PARP have been described as nuclear proteins that are involved in nucleic acid metabolism, modulation of chromatin structure, DNA synthesis, and DNA repair [51, 52]. PARP also auto-modifies itself in the presence of DNA strand breaks and is one of the main acceptors of poly(ADP-ribose) *in vivo*. PARP1 is the founding member and best-characterized member of the PARP family. PARP1 is a 116 kDa DNA repair enzyme with nuclear concentrations ranging from 2×10^5 to 1×10^6 enzymes/nucleus in eukaryotic cells [53]. PARP1 has a modular domain architecture that associates DNA damage detection with poly(ADP-ribosyl)ation activity [54]. Within 30 seconds of the advent of DNA damage, PARP1 poly(ADP-ribosyl)ates (PARylates) itself, activating the enzyme and leading to a 500-fold increase in its activity over basal levels [55]. PARP2 is most closely related to PARP1 with 69% similarity in its catalytic domain and was identified on the basis of the persistence of PARP activity in PARP1-deficient cells.

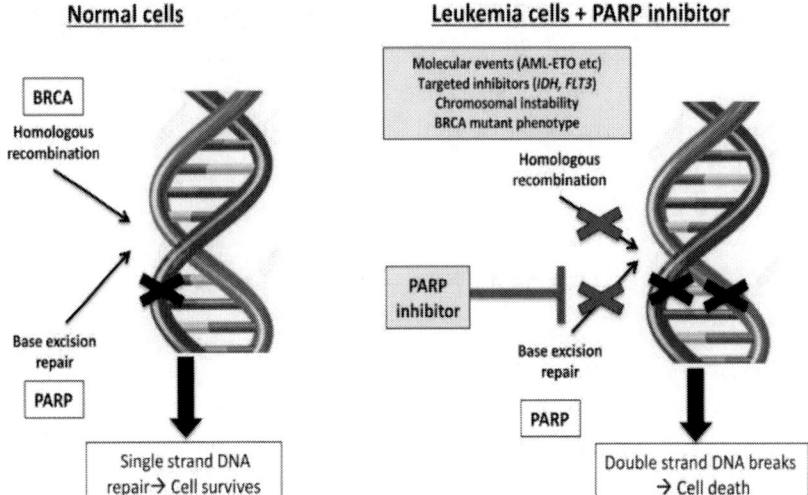

Figure 2. PARP inhibitor functions as a competitive inhibitor of nicotinamide adenine dinucleotide (NAD+) at the catalytic site of PARP1 and PARP2 enzymes. These enzymes are induced by single-strand breaks (SSBs) of the damaged DNA and are involved in the base excision repair (BER) pathway. Inhibition of the BER pathway by PARP inhibitor leads to the accumulation of unpaired SSBs, which leads to the formation of deleterious double-strand breaks (DSBs) [37]. In cells with an intact homologous recombination repair deficiencies, PARP inhibitor causes synthetic lethality through the combination of two molecular events that are otherwise nonlethal when occuring in isolation.

Four members of the PARP family (PARP1, PARP2, PARP5A, and PARP5B) can synthesize PAR chains [56-58]. The remaining members of the PARP family share the ability to bind NAD and transfer ADP-ribose groups, although some are mono(ADP-ribosyl) transferases [59, 60].

PARP1 AND ITS ROLE IN SINGLE-STRAND BREAKS REPAIR

Single strand breaks (SSBs) are directly created through cleavage of the ribose-phosphate backbone by oxidants, free radicals, radiation, or by enzymatic cleavage of DNA by topoisomerase 1 poisons. SSBs can be also formed indirectly following the excision of damaged bases by glycosylases and cleavage of the excision site by an endonuclease [61, 62]. Damaged bases are those that are methylated or oxidized. DNA-binding domain of the PARP1 recognizes the SSB. DNA binding domain contains three zinc-finger motifs. A conformational change after the binding of this zinc-finger motif 2 to the DNA activates PARP1 to cleave NAD+ into nicotinamide and an ADP-ribose moiety. The ADP-ribose group is then bound to either PARP1 or other nuclear proteins, such as histones. Other ADP-ribose groups are additionally added to the first ADP-ribose group forming negatively charged polymer. The DNA repair protein XRCC1 is recruited to the site of the break and causes the PARylated histones and PARP1 to dissociate from the break site through electrostatic repulsion. Two enzymes, poly(ADP-ribose) glycohydrolase (PARG) and ADP-ribosylhydrolase 3 (ARH3) play a central role in the degradation of PAR through their exoglycosidic and endoglycosidic activities. Digestion of PAR allows histones to reassociate with DNA and allows PARP1 to attach to other breaks and start the SSB repair in another location [63, 64].

INHIBITION OF DNA REPAIR BY PARP INHIBITORS THROUGH PARP TRAPPING

PARP trapping refers to the prevention of PARP1dissociation from the DNA in the presence of PARP inhibitor. When DNA damage occurs in the presence of a PARP inhibitor, PARP1 binds to damage sites and remains tightly bound or trapped onto the chromatin. PARylation is inhibited, and PARP1 remains bound to the lesion. The result of this trapping is replication fork collapse and DNA-double breaks which are repaired in homologous recombination-competent cells. However, in homologous recombination - defective cells, this effect is cytotoxic. PARP inhibitors trap PARP onto damaged chromatin. PARP trapping has an important effect on the tolerability and efficacy of PARP inhibitors in monotherapy situations. The PARP inhibitor-induced trapping drives single-agent cytotoxicity also in healthy human bone marrow, indicating that the toxicity of trapped PARP complexes is not restricted to malignant cells with homologous recombination deficiency [65]. The inverse relationship between trapping potency and tolerability may limit the potential therapeutic advantage of potent trapping activity.

Studies have shown that PARP inhibitors with similar catalytic activity inhibition potency can differ in their ability to induce PARP1 trapping [66, 67]. The difference in trapping potency between talazoparib and other PARP inhibitors is up to 10,000-fold, whereas catalytic potency only differs up to 40-fold. The trapping potency may not have a significant effect on the monotherapy activity of PARP inhibitors in the clinic. The concentration of PARP inhibitors necessary for the bone marrow toxicity is multiple times higher than that required to inhibit PARP synthesis. However, this trapping potency which is a key driver of bone marrow toxicity may be important for combination regimens that also induce bone marrow toxicity [65].

PRECLINICAL STUDIES OF PARP INHIBITOR OLAPARIB IN MDS AND AML CELLS

The microsatellite instability present in MDS/AML patients correlated with the down-regulation of homologous recombination repair genes [68]. Monoallelic mutations in C-terminal binding protein–interacting protein (CtIP) and double-strand-specific 3'-5' exonuclease activity of double-strand break repair protein MRE11, a component of the MRN complex necessary for double-strand repair by homologous recombination, contribute to the sensitivity of MDS/AML cells to PARP inhibitors [68].

Freshly isolated primary bone marrow cells of 28 adults with newly diagnosed MDS and one patient with low-blast count AML were cultured for 7 days with olaparib alone and with olaparib in combination with hypomethylating agent-decitabine [69]. Apoptosis in primary MDS cells was measured using an annexin-V apoptosis kit, and analyzed by flow cytometry. Fluorochrome-tagged monoclonal antibodies for differentiation markers were used for immunophenotype analysis. Olaparib favored the maturation of myeloid cells toward the neutrophilic lineage, as shown by the induction of myeloid-specific transcription factors and increased levels of metamyelocytes and neutrophils.

Mouse primary hematopoietic cells transformed by RUNX1-RUNXT1were especially sensitive to PARP inhibitors olaparib and veliparib in comparison with normal bone marrow [70]. Low expression of genes associated with homologous recombination, including RAD51, ATM (ataxia telangiectasia mutated), BRCA1, BRCA2, correlated with PARP inhibitors cytotoxicity. Recurrent IDH1 and IDH2 mutations occur in about 20% of patients with AML and 5% of patients with MDS [71-73]. Several studies showed that *IDH1* and *IDH2* mutations caused increased DNA damage, impaired homologous recombination, and increased sensitization to daunorubicin, irradiation, and the PARP inhibitors in cancer cells including AML cells [74-76].

FLT3-ITD AML has high genomic instability via overexpression of the alternative end-joining (Alt-EJ) repair pathway factors LIG3 (DNA ligase 3) and PARP1 caused by the induction of MYC expression [77-80]. These findings are in agreement with reports showing that MYC-dependent Burkitt lymphoma, neuroblastoma, and multiple myeloma are sensitive to PARP inhibition [81-83]. In addition, cells expressing *FLT3-ITD* display increased ROS production and stimulate inter-chromosomal homologous recombination. The result of these processes is loss of heterozygosity which is often found in myeloid malignancies [84, 85]. Inhibition of FLT3-ITD activity by tyrosine kinase inhibitor quizartinib (AC220) decreased homologous recombination and the alternative end-joining non-homogenous (Alt-NHEJ) repair pathway protein expression (Figure 3) [86-88].

Histone deacetylase (HDAC) inhibitors also sensitize AML cells to PARP inhibitors (Figure 3) [89, 90]. Therefore, the combination of HDAC inhibitor and PARP inhibitor showed a synergistic effect [91, 92]. Gaymes et al. demonstrated that HDAC inhibitor, entinostat (MS275), enhanced the cytotoxic effect of the PARP inhibitor KU-0058948 in leukemic cells *in vitro* [91]. Combinatorial effects of PARP inhibitor PJ34 and histone deacetylase inhibitor vorinostat on leukemia cell lines were described [92].

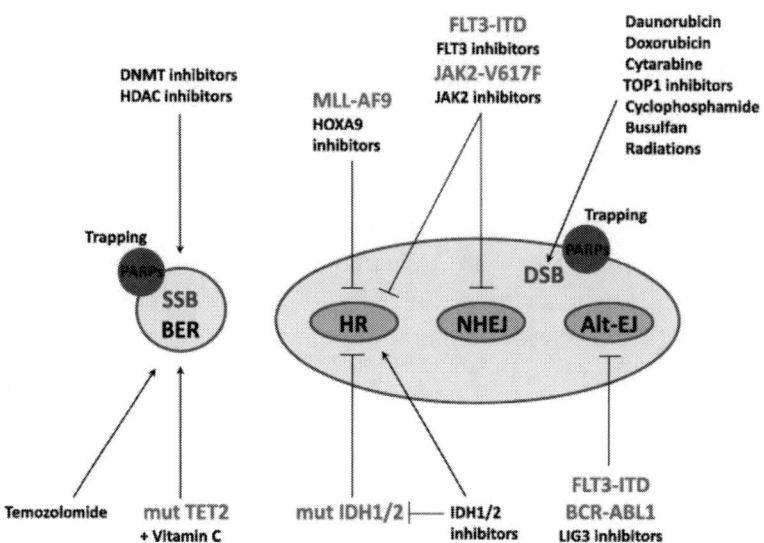

Figure 3. Combination therapies with the goal to increase activity and potency of PARP inhibitors. DNMT inhibitors, HDAC inhibitors, and temozolomide increased single strand breaks and sensitized PARP inhibitors. IDH1/2 inhibitors antagonized PARP inhibitors, since they restored ATM expression and decreased DNA damage. FLT3 inhibitors synergize PARP inhibitors [88]. Abbreviations: BER-base excision repair; SSB-single strand break; HR-homologous recombination; NHEJ-non homologous end joining; Alt-EJ-alternative NHEJ; mut-mutated; LIG-3-ATP-dependent DNA ligase 3; DNMT-DNA methyltransferase; HDAC-histone deacetylase; TET2-the ten-eleven translocation-2 gene encoding Tet methylcytosine dioxygenase 2.

PARP inhibitors also synergizes with hypomethylating agents (azacitidine and decitabine). Reactivation of hypermethylated tumor suppressors and induction of DNA damage is the main mechanism of action of these drugs. Base excision repair recognizes the lesions induced by decitabine [93]. The combination of decitabine plus olaparib resulted in a synergistic elevation in single-strand breaks and synthetic lethality since it prevented the DNA repair protein XRCC1 relocation to DNA damage sites, disrupted XRCC1-DNMT1/DNA (cytosine-5)-methyltransferase 1/co-localization, and hindered the base excision repair [93]. Other studies with combinations of low doses of hypomethylating agents (azacitidine or decitabine) and PARP inhibitors (talazoparib or olaparib), induced also synergistic cytotoxic effects in AML cells. These combinations of drugs increased DNA damage and hampered DNA repair [94, 95].

The *in vitro* combination of gemtuzumab ozogamicin, an anti-CD33 humanized monoclonal antibody linked to calicheamicin, with olaparib exhibited synergistic cytotoxicity in CD33-positive HL-60 AML cells [96]. Olaparib was also much more effective in combination with a novel CD33-targeting antibody-drug conjugated to a DNA methylating agent (IMGN779) [97]. This combination increased apoptosis, reduced cell viability, and induced almost complete S-phase cell cycle arrest. The combination of olaparib with IMGN779 significantly decreased leukemic burden and improved overall survival in human CD33+ AML xenografts [97].

Table 1. Clinical trials with PARP inhibitors in AML and MDS

Trial Identification	Disease	Phase	Drugs
NCT01399840	AML, MDS, CLL, MCL	1 dose escalation study	talazoparib
NCT01139970	R/R AML, secondary AML, CMML, or newly diagnosed AML, age>60 years with high risk features	1 dose escalation study	veliparib plus temozolomide
NCT00588991	R/R AML, high-risk MDS, aggressive MPN and CMML	1 dose escalation study	veliparib plus topotecan plus carboplatin
NCT03289910	primary AML, R/R AML, secondary AML	2	veliparib plus topotecan plus carboplatin
NCT02878785	previously untreated AML patients unfit for cytotoxic chemotherapy (arm A)	1 dose finding	talazoparib plus decitabine
	R/R AML (arm B)		
	R/R AML previously treated with decitabine, azacitidine or guadecitabine	2 based on phase 1 data	

Abbreviations: CLL-chronic lymphocytic leukemia, MCL-mantle cell lymphoma, CMML-chronic myelomonocytic leukemia, MPN- myeloproliferation

CLINICAL STUDIES WITH PARP INHIBITORS IN MDS AND AML

A phase 1 clinical trial (NCT01399840) determined the maximum tolerated dose of talazoparib in patients with advanced AML, MDS, CLL, and MCL (Table 1). Veliparib has been studied and evaluated in two combinatorial regimens in AML patients. The phase 1 study (NCT01139970) has evaluated escalating doses of veliparib plus temozolomide in 48 patients with relapsed/refractory AML, secondary AML, CMML, or newly diagnosed AML (Table 1) [98]. Temozolomide is an alkylating agent used as a treatment for some brain cancers. It was used as a second-line treatment for astrocytoma and as a first-line treatment for glioblastoma. High-risk AML patients received temozolomide 200 mg/m^2 per day for 7 days along with veliparib 150 mg twice daily for 9 days. Complete responses were reached in 8 of 48 patients (16.6%). Seven patients from this group of eight patients with complete response achieved complete response after a single cycle of the treatment. Further 8 patients achieved stable disease or hematologic improvement. Five patients received an allogeneic transplant of hematopoietic stem cells and three of these five patients were in remission after study treatment. Responders exhibited a veliparib-induced increase in histone H2AX phosphorylation in CD34+ cells, and 3 of 4 patients with the O^6-methylguanine-DNA methyltransferase (*MGMT*) gene promoter methylation achieved complete remission [98]. *MGMT* is located on chromosome 10q26.3 and encodes ubiquitously expressed enzyme involved in DNA repair [99, 100].

Veliparib has also been studied in combination with topotecan and carboplatin in patients with AML [101]. Veliparib was administered orally twice daily with dose escalation. Topotecan and carboplatin were administered together by intravenous infusion over 120 h on days 3-7 of each cycle. The total number of patients was 99 (34 patients with primary refractory AML, 35 patients with secondary AML, 22 patients with aggressive CMML or AML arising out of CMML, and 4 with refractory ALL). Response to the treatment was found in 33% of patients (14 complete remissions, 11 complete remissions with incomplete hematologic recovery, and 8 partial responses) [101].

Based on these results, a phase II trial (NCT03289910) of veliparib 80 mg twice a day plus fixed-dose carboplatin and topotecan in patients with newly diagnosed relapsed/refractory AML has been started (Table 1). Only 12 patients were recruited over six years because carboplatin and topotecan are not standard regimens for AML therapy.

SELECTIVE PARP1 DEGRADATION AVOID PARP1 TRAPPING

Cancers bearing mutations in *BRCA1* and *BRCA2* are deficient for homologous recombination. These tumors rely on PARP1 for genome integrity and are very sensitive to PARP inhibitors. This mechanism was called synthetic lethality [102, 103]. PARP inhibitors block PARP synthesis and may also kill tumor cells using a trapping mechanism [66]. Auto-PARylation of PARP1 is associated with its dissociation from DNA. The treatment with PARP inhibitors prevents auto-PARylation of PARP1 and causes its trapping at DNA lesions. This complex of PARP1, PARP inhibitor, and DNA interferes with subsequent DNA replication and therefore is highly cytotoxic [104].

Recently, targeted PARP1 protein degradation using Proteolysis Targeting Chimeras (PROTACs) has emerged as a non-trapping way for the inhibition of the growth of cancer cells bearing *BRCA 1/2* mutation and non-oncological diseases driven by aberrant PARP1 activation [105-110]. PROTACs induce potent and specific degradation of PARP1 in cancer cells at low picomolar concentrations and can be used as a single agent or in combination with cytotoxic agents, such as temozolomide and cisplatin. Up to now, PARP1 PROTACs have not been studied in AML cells. PARP1 is aberrantly activated in many non-oncological diseases, leading to excessive NAD+ depletion and PAR formation. This PARP1 activation caused cell death and tissue damage. PARP1 depletion induced by the PROTACs offered a profound protective effect in the relevant animal models.

CONCLUSION

Poly(ADP-ribose) polymerase (PARP) inhibitors induce synthetic lethality in BRCA-mutant breast and ovarian cancers [111]. Cancers bearing mutations in *BRCA1* and *BRCA2* are deficient for homologous recombination and become selectively vulnerable to PARP inhibitors. PARP inhibitors emerged as a novel therapeutic approach for AML. This is based on the fact that AML subtypes express a "BRCAness" phenotype or have genetic aberrations such as *RUNX1-RUNXT1, IDH1/2,* and *FLT3* mutations affecting DNA damage repair. To date, PARP inhibitors have exhibited limited single activity but have been very tolerable in clinical studies. Combination regimens with hypomethylating agents, histone deacetylase inhibitors, *FLT3* inhibitors in *FLT3* mutant AML, or cytotoxic agents, were more efficient. Recently, potent degraders of PARP1 were developed on the basis of PROTAC degraders. These compounds induce potent and specific degradation of PARP1 in various human cancer cells even at low picomolar concentrations when used as a single agent or in combination with cytotoxic agents.

ACKNOWLEDGMENTS

This work was supported by the project for conceptual development of research organization No 00023736 (Institute of Hematology and Blood Transfusion) from the Ministry of Health of the Czech Republic.

REFERENCES

[1] Bejar, R; Steensma, DP. Recent developments in myelodysplastic syndromes. *Blood.*, 2014, 124, 2793-2803.
[2] Pellagatti, A; Boultwood, J. The molecular pathogenesis of the myelodysplastic syndromes. *Eur. J. Haematol.*, 2015, 95, 3-15.

[3] Shastri, A; Will, B; Steidl, U; Verma, A. Stem and progenitor cell alterations in myelodysplastic syndromes. *Blood.*, 2017, 129, 1586-1594.

[4] Nazha, A; Sekeres, MA. Precision medicine in myelodysplastic syndromes and leukemias: Lessons from sequential mutations. *Annu. Rev. Med.*, 2017, 68, 127-137.

[5] Nazha, A. The MDS genomics-prognosis symbiosis. *Hematology. American Society of Hematology Education Program.*, 2018, 2018, 270-276.

[6] Barreyro, L; Chlon, TM; Starczynowski, DT. Chronic immune response dysregulation in MDS pathogenesis. *Blood.*, 2018, 132, 1553-1560.

[7] Germing, U; Schroeder, T; Kaivers, J; Kundgen, A; Kobbe, G; Gattermann, N. Novel therapies in low- and high-risk myelodysplastic syndrome. *Expert Rev. Hematol.*, 2019, 12, 893-908.

[8] Platzbecker, U; Kubasch, AS; Homer-Bouthiette, C; Prebet, T. Current challenges and unmet medical needs in myelodysplastic syndromes. *Leukemia.*, 2021, doi: 10.1038/s41375-021-01265-7.

[9] Li, L; Yang, L; Zhang, Y; Xu, Z; Qin, T; Hao, Y; Xiao, Z. Detoxification and DNA repair genes polymorphisms and susceptibility of primary myelodysplastic syndromes in Chinese population. *Leuk. Res.*, 2011, 35, 762-765.

[10] Zhou, T; Chen, P; Gu, J; Bishop, AJ; Scott, LM; Hasty, P; Rebel, VI. Potential relationship between inadequate response to DNA damage and development of myelodysplastic syndrome. *Int. J. Mol. Sci.*, 2015, 16, 966-989.

[11] Ribeiro, HL; Jr. de Oliveira, RT; Maia, AR; Pires Ferreira Filho, LI; de Sousa, JC; Heredia, FF; et al. Polymorphisms of DNA repair genes are related to the pathogenesis of myelodysplastic syndrome. *Hematol. Oncol.*, 2015, 33, 220-228.

[12] Zhang, X; Yuan, X; Zhu, W; Qian, H; Xu, W. SALL4: an emerging cancer biomarker and target. *Cancer Lett.*, 2015, 357, 55-62.

[13] Wang, F; Gao, C; Lu, J; Tatetsu, H; Williams, DA; Műller, LU; et al. Leukemic survival factor SALL4 contributes to defective DNA damage repair. *Oncogene.*, 2016, 35, 6087-6095.

[14] Valka, J; Vesela, J; Votavova, H; Dostalova-Merkerova, M; Horakova, Z; Campr, V; et al. Differential expression of homologous recombination DNA repair genes in the early and advanced stages of myelodysplastic syndrome. *Eur. J. Haematol.*, 2017, 99, 323-331.

[15] Ribeiro, HL; Jr. Maia, ARS; de Oliveira, RT; Costa, MB; Farias, IR; de Paula Borges, D; et al. DNA repair gene expressions are related to bone marrow cellularity in myelodysplastic syndrome. *J. Clin. Pathol.*, 2017, 70, 970-980.

[16] Ribeiro, HL; Jr. Maia, ARS; de Oliveira, RT; Dos Santos, AWA; Costa, MB; Farias, IR; et al. Expression of DNA repair genes is important molecular findings in CD34+ stem cells of myelodysplastic syndrome. *Eur. J. Haematol.*, 2018, 100, 108-109.

[17] Ribeiro, HL; Jr. de Oliveira, RT; de Paula Borges, D; Costa, MB; Farias, IR; Dos Santos, AWA; et al. Can synthetic lethality approach be used with DNA repair genes for primary and secondary MDS? *Med. Oncol.*, 2019, 36, 99.

[18] Aly, M; Ramdzan, ZM; Nagata, Y; Balasubramanian, SK; Hosono, N; Makishima, H; et al. Distinct clinical and biological implications of CUX1 in myeloid neoplasms. *Blood Adv.*, 2019, 3, 2164-2178.

[19] Swelem, RS; Elneely, DA; Shehata, AAR. The study of SALL4 gene and BMI-1 gene expression in acute myeloid leukemia patients. *Lab. Med.*, 2020, 51, 265-270.

[20] Imgruet, MK; Lutze, J; An, N; Hu, B; Khan, S; Kurkewich, J; et al. Loss of a 7q gene, *CUX1*, disrupts epigenetic-driven DNA repair and drives therapy-related myeloid neoplasms. *Blood.*, 2021, doi: 10.1182/blood. 2020009195.

[21] Schanz, J; Cevik, N; Fonatsch, C; Braulke, F; Shirneshan, K; Bacher, U; Haase, D. Detailed analysis of clonal evolution and cytogenetic evolution patterns in patients with myelodysplastic syndromes (MDS)and related myeloid disorders. *Blood Cancer J.*, 2018, 8, 28.

[22] Esposito, MT; So, CW. DNA damage accumulation and repair defects in acute myeloid leukemia: implications for pathogenesis, disease progression, and chemotherapy resistance. *Chromosoma.*, 2014, 123, 545-561.

[23] Popp, HD; Naumann, N; Brendel, S; Henzler, T; Weiss, C; Hofmann, WK; Fabarius, A. Increase of DNA damage and alteration of the DNA damage response in myelodysplastic syndromes and acute myeloid leukemias. *Leuk. Res.*, 2017, 57, 112-118.

[24] Wong, TN; Miller, CA; Jotte, MRM; Bagegni, N; Baty, JD; Schmidt, AP; et al. Cellular stressors contribute to the expansion of hematopoietic clones of varying leukemic potential. *Nat. Commun.*, 2018, 9, 455.

[25] Hsu, JI; Dayaram, T; Tovy, A; de Braekeleer, E; Jeong, M; Wang, F; et al. PPM1D mutations drive clonal hematopoiesis in response to cytotoxic chemotherapy. *Cell Stem Cell.*, 2018, 23, 700-713.

[26] Ok, CY; Patel, KP; Garcia-Manero, G; Routbort, MJ; Peng, J; Tang, G; et al. TP53 mutation chaacteristics in therapy-related myelodysplastic syndromes and acute myeloid leukemia is similar to de novo diseases. *J. Hematol. Oncol.*, 2015, 8, 45.

[27] Wong, TN; Ramsingh, G; Young, AL; Miller, CA; Touma, W; Welch, JS; et al. Role of TP53 mutations in the origin and evolution of therapy-related acute myeloid leukaemia. *Nature.*, 2015, 518, 552-555.

[28] Welch, S. Patterns of mutations in TP53 mutated AML. *Best Pract. Res. Clin. Haematol.*, 2018, 31, 379-383.

[29] Barbosa, K; Li, S; Adams, PD; Desphande, AJ. The role of TP53 in acute myeloid leukemia: challenges and opportunities. *Genes Chromosomes Cancer.*, 2019, 58, 875-888.

[30] Britt, A; Mohyuddin, GR; McClune, B; Singh, A; Lin, T; Ganguly, S; et al. Acute myeloid leukemia or myelodysplastic syndrome with chromosome 17 abnormalities and long-term outcomes with or without hematopoietic stem cell transplantation. *Leuk. Res.*, 2020, 95, 106402.

[31] Molicce, M; Mazzone, C; Niscola, P; de Fabritis, P. *TP53* mutations in acute myeloid leukemia: still a daunting challenge? *Front. Oncol.*, 2021, 10, 610820.

[32] Pearsall, EA; Lincz, LF; Skelding, KA. The role of DNA repair pathways in AML chemosensitivity. *Curr. Drug Targets.*, 2018, 19, 1205-1219.

[33] Dulaney, C; Marcrom, S; Stanley, J; Yang, ES. Poly(ADP-ribose) polymerase activity and inhibition in cancer. *Semin. Cell Dev. Biol.*, 2017, 63, 144-153.

[34] Curtin, NJ; Szabo, C. Poly(ADP-ribose) polymerase inhibition: past, present and future. *Nat. Rev. Drug Discov.*, 2020, 19, 711-736.

[35] Amé, JC; Spenlehauer, C; de Murcia, G. The PARP superfamily. *BioEssays.*, 2004, 26, 882-893.

[36] Murai, J; Huang, SN; Das, BB; Renaud, A; Zhang, Y; Doroshow, JH; et al. Trapping of PARP1 and PARP2 by clinical PARP inhibitors. *Cancer Res.*, 2012, 72, 5588-5599.

[37] Fritz, C; Portwood, SM; Przespolewski, A; Wang, ES. PARP goes the weasel! Emerging role of PARP inhibitors in acute leukemias. *Blood Rev.*, 2021, 45, 100696.

[38] de Murcia, JM; Niedergang, C; Trucco, C; Ricoul, M; Dutrillaux, B; Mark, M; et al. Requirement of poly(ADP-ribose) polymerase in recovery from DNA damage in mice and in cells. *Proc. Natl. Acad. Sci. U.S.A.*, 1997, 94, 7303–7307.

[39] Trucco, C; Oliver, FJ; de Murcia, G; Ménissier-de Murcia, J. DNA repair defect in poly(ADP-ribose) polymerase-deficient cell lines. *Nucleic Acids Res.*, 1998, 26, 2644–2649.

[40] Javle, M; Curtin, NJ. The role of PARP in DNA repair and its therapeutic exploitation. *Br. J. Cancer.*, 2011, 105, 1114–1122.

[41] De Vos, M; Schreiber, V; Dantzer, F. The diverse roles and clinical relevance of PARPs in DNA damage repair: current state of the art. *Biochem. Pharmacol.*, 2012, 84, 137–146.

[42] Amé, JC; Rolli, V; Schreiber, V; Niedergang, C; Apiou, F; Decker, P; et al. PARP-2, a novel mammalian DNA damage-dependent poly(ADP-ribose) polymerase. *J. Biol. Chem.*, 1999, 274, 17860–17868.

[43] Schreiber, V; Amé, JC; Dollé, P; Schultz, I; Rinaldi, B; Fraulob, V; et al. Poly(ADP-ribose) polymerase-2 (PARP-2) is required for efficient base excision DNA repair in association with PARP-1 and XRCC1. *J. Biol. Chem.*, 2002, 277, 23028–23036.

[44] Yélamos, J; Schreiber, V; Dantzer, F. Toward specific functions of poly(ADP-ribose) ppolymerase-2. *Trends Mol. Med.*, 2008, 14, 169–178.

[45] Szabo, C; Zingarelli, B; O´Connor, M; Salzman, AL. DNA strand breakage, activation of poly(ADP-ribose)synthetase, and cellular energy depletion are involved in the cytotoxicity of macrophages and smooth muscle cells exposed to peroxynitrite. *Proc. Natl. Acad. Sci. U.S.A.*, 1996, 93, 1753–1758.

[46] Virag, L; Salzman, AL; Szabo, C. Poly(ADP-ribose) synthetase activation mediates mitochondrial injury during oxidant-induced cell death. *J. Immunol.*, 1998, 161, 3753-3759.

[47] Andrabi, SA; Kim, NS; Yu, SW; Wang, H; Koh, DW; Sasaki, M; et al. Poly(ADP-ribose) (PAR) polymer is a death signal. *Proc. Natl. Acad. Sci. U.S.A.*, 2006, 103, 18308–18313.

[48] Heeres, JT; Hergenrother, PJ. Poly(ADP-ribose) makes a date with death. *Curr. Opin. Chemical Biol.*, 2007, 11, 644–653.

[49] Krishnakumar, R; Kraus, WL. PARP-1 regulates chromatin structure and transcription through a KDM5B-dependent pathway. *Mol. Cell.*, 2010, 39, 736–749.

[50] Kraus, WL; Hottiger, MO. PARP-1 and gene regulation: progress and puzzles. *Mol. Aspects Med.*, 2013, 34, 1109–1123.

[51] Poirier, GG; de Murcia, G; Jongstra-Bilen, J; Niedergang, C; Mandel, P. Poly(ADP-ribosyl)ation of polynucleosomes causes relaxation of chromatin structure. *Proc. Natl. Acad. Sci. U.S.A.*, 1982, 79, 3423–3427.

[52] Gottschalk, AJ; Timinszky, G; Kong, SE; Jin, J; Cai, Y; Swanson, SK; et al. Poly(ADP-ribosyl)ation directs recruitment and activation of an ATP-dependent chromatin remodeler. *Proc. Natl. Acad. Sci. U.S.A.*, 2009, 106, 13770–13774.

[53] Ludwig, A; Behnke, B; Hotlund, J; Hilz, H. Immunoquantitation and size determination of intrinsic poly(ADP-ribose) polymerase from acid precipitates. An analysis of the *in vivo* status in mammalian species and in lower eukaryotes. *J. Biol. Chem.* 1988, 263, 6993-6999.

[54] Langelier, MF; Planck, JL; Roy, S; Pascal, JM. Structural basis for DNA-dependent poly (ADP-ribosyl)ation by human PARP-1. *Science.*, 2012, 336, 728-732.

[55] Herceg, Z; Wang, ZQ. Functions of poly (ADP-ribose) polymerase (PARP) in DNA repair, genomic integrity and cell death. *Mutat. Res.*, 2001, 477, 97-110.

[56] Gibson, BA; Kraus, WL. New insights into the molecular and cellular functions of poly(ADP-ribose) and PARPS. *Nat. Rev. Mol. Cell Biol.*, 2012, 13, 411-424.

[57] Kraus, WL. PARPs and ADP-ribosylation: 50 years and counting. *Mol. Cell.*, 2015, 58, 902-910.

[58] Cohen, MS; Chang, P. Insights into the biogenesis, function, and regulation of ADP-ribosylation. *Nat. Chem. Biol.*, 2018, 14, 236-245.

[59] Rouleau, M; Patel, A; Hendzel, MJ; Kaufmann, SH; Poirier, GG. PARP inhibition: PARP1 and beyond. *Nat. Rev. Cancer.*, 2010, 10, 293–301.

[60] Hassa, PO; Hottiger, MO. The diverse biological roles of mammalian PARPS, a small but powerful family of poly-ADP-ribose polymerases. *Front. Biosci.*, 2008, 13, 3046–3082.

[61] Parsons, JL; Dianov, GL. Co-ordination of base excision repair and genome stability. *DNA Repair.*, 2013, 12, 326-333.

[62] Krokan, HE; Bjorås, M. Base excision repair. *Cold Spring Harb. Perspect. Biol.*, 2013, 5, a012583.

[63] Caldecott, KW. Protein ADP-ribosylation and the cellular response to DNA strand breaks. *DNA Repair.*, 2014, 19, 108-113.

[64] Martin-Hernandez, K; Rodriguez-Vargas, JM; Schreiber, V; Dantzer, F. Expanding functions of ADP-ribosylation in the maintenance of genome integrity. *Semin. Cell Dev. Biol.*, 2017, 63, 92-101.

[65] Hopkins, TA; Ainsworth, WB; Ellis, PA; Donawho, CK; DiGiammarino, L; Panchal, SC; et al. *Mol. Cancer Res.*, 2019, 17, 409-419.

[66] Pommier, Y; O'Connor, MJ; de Bono, J. Laying a trap to kill cancer cells: PARP inhibitors and their mechanisms of action. *Sci. Transl. Med.*, 2016, 8, 362ps17.

[67] Murai, J; Huang, SY; Renaud, A; Zhang, Y; Ji, J; Takeda, S; et al. Stereospecific PARP trapping by BMN673 and comparison with olaparib and rucaparib. *Mol. Cancer Ther.*, 2014, 13, 433-443.

[68] Gaymes, TJ; Mohamedali, M; Patterson, M; Matto, N; Smith, A; Kulasekararaj, A; et al. Microsatellite instability induced mutations in DNA repair genesCtIPand MRE11 confer hypersensitivity to

poly (ADP-ribose) polymerase inhibitors in myeloid malignancies. *Haematologica.*, 2013, 98, 1397-1406.

[69] Faraoni, I; Consalvo, MI; Aloisio, F; Fabiani, E; Giansanti, M; Di Cristino, F; et al. Cytotoxicity and differentiating effect of the poly(ADP-Ribose) polymerase inhibitor olaparib in myelodysplastic syndromes. *Cancers.*, 2019, 11, 1373.

[70] Esposito, MT; Zhao, L; Fung, TK; Rane, JK; Wilson, A; Martin, N; et al. Synthetic lethal targeting of oncogenic transcription factors in acute leukemia by PARP inhibitors. *Nat. Med.*, 2015, 21, 1481-1490.

[71] Molenaar, RJ; Thota, S; Nagata, Y; Patel, B; Clemente, M; Hirsh, C; et al. Clinical and biological implications of ancestral and non-ancestral IDH1 and IDH2 mutations in myeloid neoplasms. *Leukemia.*, 2015, 29, 2134-2142.

[72] DiNardo, C; Jabbour, E; Ravandi, F; Takahashi, K; Daver, N; Routbort, M; et al. IDH1 and IDH2 mutations in myelodysplastic syndromes and role in disease progression. *Leukemia.*, 2016, 30, 980-984.

[73] Marcucci, G; Maharry, K; Wu, YZ; Radmacher, MD; Mrózek, K; Margeson, D; et al. *IDH1* and *IDH2* gene mutations identify novel molecular subsets within de novo cytogenetically normal acute myeloid leukemia: a cancer and leukemia group B study. *J. Clin. Oncol.*, 2010, 28, 2348-2355.

[74] Molenaar, RJ; Radivoyevitch, T; Nagata, Y; Khurshed, M; Przychodzen, B; Makishima, H; et al. *IDH1/2* mutations sensitize acute myeloid leukemia to PARP inhibition and this is reversed by IDH1/2-mutant inhibitors. *Clin. Cancer Res.*, 2018, 24, 1705-1715.

[75] Sulkowski, PL; Corso, CD; Robinson, ND; Scanlon, SE; Purshouse, KR; Bai, H; et al. 2-hydroxyglutarate produced neomorphic IDH mutations suppresses homologous recombination and induces PARP inhibitor sensitivity. *Sci. Transl. Med.*, 2017, 9, eaal2463.

[76] Megías-Vericat, JE; Ballesta-López, O; Barragán, E; Montesinos, P. IDH1-mutated relapsed or refractory AML: current challenges and future prospects. *Blood Lymphat. Cancer.*, 2019, 9, 19-32.

[77] Fan, J; Li, L; Small, D; Rassool, F. Cells expressing FLT3/ITD mutations exhibit elevated repair errors generated through

alternative NHEJ pathways: implications for genomic instability and therapy. *Blood.*, 2010, 116, 5298-5305.

[78] Muvarak, N; Kelley, S; Robert, C; Baer, MR; Perrotti, D; Gambacorti-Passerini, C; et al. c –MYC generates repair errors via increased transcription of alternative NHEJ factors, LIG3 and PARP1, in tyrosine kinase-activated leukemias. *Mol. Cancer Res.*, 2015, 13, 699-712.

[79] Li, Z; Owonikoko, TK; Sun, SY. c-Myc suppression of DNA double-strand break repair. *Neoplasia.*, 2012, 14, 1190-1202.

[80] Karlsson, A; Deb-Basu, D; Cherry, A; Turner, S; Ford, J; Felsher, DW. Deffective double-strand DNA break repair and chromosomal translocations by MYC overexpression. *Proc. Natl. Acad. Sci. U.S.A.*, 2003, 100, 9971-9979.

[81] Maifrede, S; Martin, K; Podszywalow-Bartnicka, P. IGH/MYC translocation associates with BRCA2 deficiency and synthetic lethality to PARP1 inhibitors. *Mol. Cancer Res.*, 2017, 15, 967-972.

[82] Colicchia, V; Petroni, M; Guarguaglini, G. PARP inhibitors enhance replication stress and cause mitotic catastrophe in MYCN-dependent neuroblastoma. *Oncogene.*, 2017, 36, 4682-4691.

[83] Caracciolo, D; Scionti, F; Juli, G; Altomare, E; Golino, G; Todoerti, K; et al. Exploiting MYC-induced PARPness to target genomic instability in multiple myeloma. *Haematologica.*, 2021, 106, 185-195.

[84] Salimyr, A; Fan, J; Datta, K; Kim, KT; Grosu, D; Shapiro, P; et al. Internal tandem duplication of FLT3 (FLT3/ITD) induced increased ROS production, DNA damage, amd misrepair: implications for poor prognosis in AML. *Blood.*, 2008, 111, 3173-3182.

[85] Gaymes, TJ; Mohademali, A; Eilizadeh, Al; Darling, D; Mufti, GJ. FLT3 and JAK2 mutations in acute myeloid leukemia promote interchromosomal homologous recombination and the potential for copy neutral loss of heterozygosity. *Cancer Res.*, 2017, 77, 1697-1708.

[86] Maifrede, S; Nieborowska-Skorska, M; Sullivan-Reed, K; Dasgupta, Y; Podszywalow-Bartnicka, P; Le, BV; et al. Tyrosine

kinase inhibitor-induced defects in DNA repair sensitize FLT3(ITD)-positive leukemia cells to PARP1 inhibitors. *Blood.*, 2018, 132, 67-77.
[87] Dellomo, AJ; Baer, MR; Rassool, FV. Partnering with PARP inhibitors in acute myeloid leukemia with FLT3-ITD. *Cancer Lett.*, 2019, 454, 171-178.
[88] Faraoni, I; Giansanti, M; Voso, MT; Lo-Coco, F; Graziani, G. Targeting ADP-ribosylation by PARP inhibitors in acute leukemia and related disorders. *Biochem. Pharmacol.*, 2019, 167, 133-148.
[89] Petruccelli, LA; DupéréRicher, D; Pettersson, F; Retrouvey, H; Skoulikas, S; Miller, WH, Jr. Vorinostat induces reactive oxygen species and DNA damage in acute myeloid leukemia cells. *PLoS One.*, 2011, 6, e20987
[90] Conti, C; Leo, E; Eichler, GS; Sordet, O; Martin, MM; Fan, A; et al. Inhibition of histone deacetylase in cancer cells slows down replication forks, activates dormant origins, and induces DNA damage. *Cancer Res.*, 2010, 70, 4470-4480.
[91] Gaymes, TJ; Shall, S; MacPherson, LJ; Twine, NJ; Lea, NC; Farzaneh, F. Inhibitors of poly ADP-ribose polymerase (PARP) induce apoptosis of myeloid leukemic cells: Potential for therapy of myeloid leukemia and myelodysplastic syndromes. *Haematologica.*, 2009, 94, 638-646.
[92] Jasek, E; Gajda, M; Lis, GJ; Jasinska, M; Litwin, JA. Combinatorial effects of PARP inhibitor Vorinostat on leukemia cell lines. *Anticancer Res.*, 2014, 34, 1849-1856.
[93] Orta, ML; Höglund, A; Calderón-Montano, JM; Dominguez, I; Burgos-Morón, E; Visnes, T; et al. The PARP inhibitor olaparib disrupts base excision repair of 5-aza-2´-deoxycytidine lesions. *Nucleic Acids Res.*, 2014, 42, 9108-9120.
[94] Muvarak, NE; Chowdhury, K; Xia, L; Robert, C; Choi, EY; Cai, Y; et al. Enhancing the cytotoxic effects of PARP inhibitors with DNA demethylating agents-a potential therapy for cancer. *Cancer Cell.*, 2016, 30, 637-650.
[95] Zhao, L; So, CWE. PARPi potentiates with current conventional therapy in MLL leukemia. *Cell Cycle.*, 2017, 16, 1861-1869.
[96] Yamauchi, T; Uzui, K; Nishi, R; Shigemi, H; Ueda, T. Gemtuzumab ozogamicin and olaparib exert synergistic

cytotoxicity in CD33-positive positive HL-60 myeloid leukemia cells. *Anticancer Res.*, 2014, 34, 5487-5494.

[97] Portwood, SM; Puchalski, RA; Walker, RM; Wang, ES. Combining IMGN779, a novel anti-CD33 antibody-drug conjugate (ADC), with the PARP inhibitor, olaparib, results in enhanced anti-tumor activity in preclinical acute myeloid leukemia (AML) models. *Blood.*, 2016, 128, 1645.

[98] Gojo, I; Beumer, JH; Pratz, KW; McDevitt, MA; Baer, MR; Blackford, AL; et al. A phase 1 study of the PARP inhibitor veliparib in combination with temozolomide in acute myeloid leukemia. *Clin. Cancer Res.*, 2017, 23, 697-706.

[99] Wick, W; Weller, M; van den Bent, M; Sanson, M; Weiler, M; von, Deimling, A; et al. MGMT testing-the challenges for biomarker-based glioma treatment. *Nat. Rev. Neurol.*, 2014, 10, 372-385.

[100] Yu, W; Zhang, L; Wei, Q; Shao, A. O6-methyjguanine-DNA-methyltransferase (MGMT): challenges and new opportunities in glioma chemotherapy. *Front. Oncol.*, 2020, 9, 1547.

[101] Pratz, KW; Rudek, MA; Gojo, I; Litzow, MR; McDevitt, MA; Ji, J; et al. A phase I study of topotecan, carboplatin and the PARP inhibitor veliparib in acute leukemias, aggressive myeloproliferative neoplasms, and chronic myelomonocytic leukemia. *Clin. Cancer Res.*, 2017, 23, 899-907.

[102] Bryant, HE; Schultz, N; Thomas, HD; Parker, KM; Flower, D; Lopez, E; et al. Specific killing of BRCA2-deficient tumours with inhibitors of poly(ADP-ribose) polymerase. *Nature.*, 2005, 434, 913-917.

[103] Farmer, H; McCabe, N; Lord, CJ; Tutt, AN; Johnson, DA; Richardson, TB; et al. Targeting the DNA repair defect in BRCA murant cells as a therapeutic strategy. *Nature.*, 2005, 434, 917-921.

[104] Lord, CJ; Ashworth, A. PARP inhibitors: synthetic lethality in the clinic. *Science.*, 2017, 355, 1152-1158.

[105] Zhao, Q; Lan, T; Su, S; Rao, Y. Induction of apoptosis in MDA-MB-231 breast cancer cells by a PARP1-targeting PROTAC small molecule. *Chem. Commun.* (Camb)., 2019, 55, 369-372.

[106] Wang, S; Han, L; Han, J; Li, P; Ding, Q; Zhang, QJ; et al. Uncoupling of PARP1 trapping and inhibition using selectuve PARP1 degradation. *Nat. Chem. Biol.*, 2019, 15, 1223-1231.

[107] Zhang, Z; Chang, X; Zhang, C; Zeng, S; Liang, M; M, a Z; et al. Identification of probe-quality degraders for poly(ADP-ribose) polymerase-1 (PARP1). *J. Enzyme Inhibition Med. Chem.* 2020, 35, 1606-1615.

[108] Cao, C; Yang, J; Chen, Y; Zhou, P; Wang, Y; Du, W; et al. Discovery of SK-575 as a highly potent and efficacious proteolysis targeting chimera degrader of PARP1 for treating cancers. *J. Med. Chem.*, 2020, 63, 11012-11033.

[109] Zheng, M; Huo, J; Gu, X; Wang, Y; Wu, C; Zhang, Q; et al. Rational design and synthesis of novel dual PROTACs for simultaneous degradation of EGFR and PARP. *J. Med. Chem.*, 2021, doi: 10.1021/acs.jmedchem.1c00649.

[110] Kim, C; Chen, C; Yu, Y. Avoid the trap: Targeting PARP1 beyond human malignancy. *Cell Chem. Biol.*, 2021, 28, 456-462.

[111] Velagapudi, UK; Patel, BA; Shao, X; Pathak, SK; Ferraris, DV; Talele, TT. Recent development in the discovery of PARP inhibitors as anticancer agents: a patent update (2016-2020). *Expert Opin. Ther. Pat.*. 2021, doi: 10.1080/13543776. 2021.1886275.

INDEX

#

2-hydroxyglutarate, viii, 33, 51, 52, 53, 55, 56, 58, 73, 75, 76, 77, 78, 79, 86, 133

A

acid, x, 7, 9, 27, 28, 54, 55, 56, 58, 114, 131
acute leukemia, 22, 37, 87, 130, 133, 135, 136
acute lymphocytic leukemia (ALL), iv, 3, 16, 26, 28, 37, 91, 97, 124
acute myelogenous leukemia, 76, 109, 110
acute myeloid leukemia (AML), v, vii, viii, ix, x, 4, 12, 13, 15, 16, 18, 23, 30, 32, 33, 35, 36, 37, 46, 51, 52, 55, 56, 59, 60, 61, 62, 63, 64, 65, 66, 67, 69, 70, 71, 73, 74, 75, 76, 78, 79, 80, 81, 82, 83, 84, 85, 86, 87, 90, 91, 99, 100, 101, 102, 106, 109, 110, 111, 113, 114, 115, 116, 120, 121, 123, 124, 125, 126, 128, 129, 133, 134, 135, 136

adenine, 53, 55, 76, 116, 118
adverse event, 63, 64, 66, 67, 91, 93, 94, 95, 96, 98, 99, 100, 101, 102
age, 8, 9, 12, 13, 16, 59, 65, 70, 73, 93, 97, 99, 100, 107, 114, 116, 123
anemia, 5, 6, 8, 17, 20, 23, 43, 63, 64, 93, 98, 99
anorexia, 91, 93, 100, 101
apoptosis, x, 28, 58, 70, 93, 96, 99, 100, 101, 111, 113, 120, 123, 135, 136
arginine, 30, 33, 35, 52, 54
ASXL1, 7, 8, 15, 23, 24, 25, 30, 32, 33, 34, 37, 47, 59, 65
autosomal dominant, 4
autosomal recessive, 4

B

BCR-ABL1, 4, 7, 8, 14, 16, 17, 19, 20, 21, 22, 23, 24, 40
bilirubin, 7, 58, 63
biochemistry, 14
biological roles, 132
biomarkers, 71, 115
biopsy, 6, 11, 18
biosynthesis, 58, 78, 79
bleeding, 3, 5, 9, 13

blood circulation, 9
blood clot, 3, 5, 13
blood plasma, 3
blood pressure, 64
blood-brain barrier, 91
bone marrow, vii, x, 1, 2, 3, 5, 6, 7, 8, 9, 10, 11, 12, 13, 14, 15, 16, 18, 22, 23, 56, 64, 68, 102, 113, 120, 121, 128
bone marrow aspiration, 6, 7, 23
bone marrow biopsy, 7, 10, 14, 23, 68
brain cancer, 124
breast cancer, 136

C

calcium, 28, 45, 76
CALR, 4, 5, 7, 8, 14, 15, 24, 25, 27, 28, 34, 42, 45
cancer cells, ix, 61, 71, 90, 91, 93, 106, 121, 125, 126, 132, 135
cancer progression, 48
cancer therapy, x, 113
cell cycle, 36, 99, 123
cell death, 28, 58, 91, 93, 96, 106, 109, 111, 117, 125, 131
cell differentiation, 47, 61, 78, 85
cell line, 36, 72, 101, 114, 121, 130, 135
cell lines, 36, 72, 101, 121, 130, 135
cell surface, 7, 27, 29, 100
chemotherapy, 61, 62, 64, 67, 68, 69, 70, 74, 85, 99, 110, 116, 123, 128, 129, 136
chromosome, ix, 11, 16, 17, 18, 19, 25, 26, 27, 29, 30, 32, 33, 34, 35, 36, 40, 53, 89, 124, 129
chronic eosinophilic leukemia (CEL), vii, 1, 4, 22, 23, 41, 42
chronic lymphocytic leukemia, ix, 90, 96, 108, 109, 123
chronic myeloid leukemia (CML), vii, 1, 4, 5, 8, 14, 16, 17, 18, 20, 23, 24, 37, 40, 41, 43, 97

chronic neutrophilic leukemia (CNL), vii, 1, 4, 23, 25, 29, 45
clinical trials, ix, 4, 8, 61, 64, 74, 86, 90, 93
combination therapy, 63, 68, 69
complete blood count, 6, 10, 23
CSF3R, 4, 25, 29, 45
cytotoxicity, x, 99, 114, 119, 121, 123, 131, 136

D

degradation, x, 114, 119, 125, 126, 137
detection, 40, 77, 82, 117
diagnostic criteria, 5, 14, 38
diarrhea, 22, 93, 100, 101
differential diagnosis, viii, 2, 7
disease progression, 30, 41, 80, 97, 128, 133
diseases, vii, 2, 3, 7, 9, 10, 22, 32, 37, 42, 46, 47, 125, 129
disorder, 5, 6, 9, 13, 14, 17, 37, 44
DNA damage, x, 71, 79, 93, 106, 113, 114, 115, 116, 117, 119, 121, 122, 126, 127, 128, 129, 130, 134, 135
DNA lesions, 125
DNA ligase, 121, 122
DNA repair, x, 32, 79, 113, 115, 116, 117, 119, 122, 124, 127, 128, 129, 130, 131, 132, 135, 136
DNA sequencing, 21
DNA strand breaks, 116, 117, 132
DNA-damage, 114
DNA-repair, 114
DNMT3A, 4, 8, 12, 23, 24, 25, 30, 33, 46, 59, 60, 65, 74, 82
driver mutation, 25, 29, 34, 80
drug resistance, viii, 34, 89, 90, 104
drugs, vii, 20, 21, 72, 73, 91, 100, 112, 122

E

eltanexor, ix, 90, 91, 102
enasidenib, viii, 52, 61, 62, 66, 67, 68, 69, 74, 85, 86
encoding, 26, 30, 52, 73, 122
environmental change, 37
enzymatic activity, 53, 73
enzyme, vii, viii, x, 7, 30, 51, 52, 53, 56, 57, 73, 76, 81, 113, 116, 117, 124
erythropoietin (EPO), 10, 11
essential thrombocythemia (ET), vii, 1, 4, 8, 13, 14, 15, 18, 23, 25, 26, 27, 28, 31, 33, 34, 37, 38, 39, 40, 42, 44, 48
eukaryotic, ix, 89, 91, 117
evolution, 39, 46, 60, 80, 81, 128, 129
excision, x, 113, 116, 118, 119, 122, 130, 132, 135
exportin 1, viii, 89, 90, 92, 93, 98, 101

F

family history, 4
family members, 26
FDA, viii, 52, 53, 61, 64, 73, 84, 93
fever, 6, 17, 22, 64
FGFR1 (fibroblast growth factor receptor 1), 22, 23
Food and Drug Administration, viii, ix, 52, 53, 90, 93
formation, 3, 5, 6, 13, 26, 33, 36, 92, 117, 118, 125
fumarate hydratase, 55
fusion, x, 16, 22, 23, 24, 40, 114

G

gene expression, 33, 57, 128
gene promoter, 124
gene regulation, 131
genes, viii, x, 2, 4, 5, 7, 14, 22, 23, 24, 25, 26, 28, 30, 33, 38, 52, 57, 59, 63, 64, 66, 73, 114, 115, 116, 117, 120, 121, 127, 128
genetic alteration, 25, 82
genetic defect, 4
genetic factors, 4, 37
genetic testing, 4, 14
genome, 55, 75, 102, 125, 132
genomic instability, x, 114, 116, 121, 134
genomics, 80, 127
glioblastoma, 52, 55, 74, 75, 124
glioblastoma multiforme, 74
glioma, 72, 74, 78, 87, 136
glucocorticoid, ix, 90, 93
glucocorticoid receptor, 93
growth, viii, ix, x, 51, 55, 72, 73, 89, 91, 113, 125

H

health care, vii, 37
health problems, 13
hematocrit, 10, 11, 12, 13, 15
hematologic malignancies, v, vii, ix, 51, 86, 89, 90, 98, 105, 109
hematopoietic stem cells, vii, 1, 3, 5, 16, 29, 36, 46, 56, 124
hemoglobin, 2, 8, 10, 11, 13, 24, 68
hepatocellular carcinoma, 48
histone, viii, 9, 33, 34, 38, 47, 51, 53, 55, 57, 58, 61, 66, 73, 77, 78, 121, 122, 124, 126, 135
histone deacetylase, 9, 121, 122, 126, 135
human, x, 2, 33, 38, 45, 46, 47, 48, 52, 53, 66, 74, 75, 76, 77, 79, 83, 100, 109, 112, 113, 119, 123, 126, 131, 137
human body, 2
human genome, 52
human leukocyte antigen, 38

hyponatremia, 93, 99, 100, 102
hypoxia-inducible factor, 57

I

IDH1, viii, 8, 12, 15, 25, 30, 32, 37, 47, 51, 52, 53, 54, 55, 56, 58, 59, 60, 61, 62, 63, 64, 65, 66, 67, 70, 71, 72, 73, 74, 75, 76, 78, 79, 80, 82, 83, 84, 85, 86, 87, 121, 122, 126, 133
IDH1 and IDH2 mutations, viii, 51, 52, 59, 60, 61, 71, 74, 75, 76, 78, 80, 82, 121, 133
IDH1/2, 8, 12, 15, 47, 83, 86, 122, 126, 133
IDH2, viii, 25, 30, 32, 51, 52, 53, 54, 55, 59, 60, 61, 66, 67, 69, 72, 73, 77, 78, 80, 81, 82, 84, 85, 121, 133
immune response, 5, 72, 80, 127
immune system, 2, 3, 7
in vitro, 28, 56, 58, 63, 91, 121, 123
in vivo, 58, 63, 75, 83, 84, 96, 117, 131
induction, 45, 61, 67, 73, 85, 100, 111, 121, 122
induction chemotherapy, 61, 68
infection, 7, 17, 18, 47, 93, 97
inhibition, 57, 58, 62, 64, 66, 70, 78, 83, 84, 86, 87, 98, 99, 101, 102, 105, 107, 108, 109, 111, 112, 120, 121, 125, 130, 132, 133, 137
inhibitor, 9, 27, 41, 58, 61, 62, 63, 64, 65, 66, 67, 72, 77, 83, 84, 85, 86, 91, 92, 94, 98, 99, 101, 103, 105, 106, 109, 110, 114, 116, 118, 119, 121, 125, 133, 135, 136
initiation, viii, ix, 2, 30, 60, 89, 91
ivosidenib, viii, 52, 61, 62, 64, 65, 67, 68, 70, 74, 84, 85, 86

J

JAK2, 4, 7, 8, 10, 11, 12, 14, 15, 22, 23, 24, 25, 26, 27, 28, 32, 33, 34, 42, 43, 44, 45, 47, 134

K

karyotype, 55, 60, 73, 97
karyotyping, 8
kidney, 7, 10, 64
kidney failure, 7, 64
kidney stones, 7
kinase activity, 17, 26
Krebs cycle, 32, 55, 56

L

leukemia, vii, ix, x, 1, 4, 6, 7, 16, 22, 24, 35, 40, 41, 42, 43, 45, 59, 61, 63, 71, 76, 79, 80, 82, 90, 99, 100, 106, 111, 114, 121, 123, 129, 133, 135, 136
ligand, x, 25, 26, 27, 29, 114
lymphoid, 16, 32, 36, 40, 42
lymphoma, ix, 22, 90, 91, 96, 97, 98, 103, 106, 108, 109, 110, 112, 121, 123
lysine, 27, 33, 34, 57, 77

M

major bcr (M-bcr), 16
major histocompatibility complex, 7, 72
marrow, 3, 5, 6, 7, 11, 14, 16, 18, 23, 71, 120
median, 5, 22, 64, 65, 66, 70, 71, 73, 94, 95, 97, 98, 99, 100, 101, 102
metabolism, 2, 56, 57, 58, 61, 117
methylation, viii, 30, 33, 34, 51, 53, 55, 57, 61, 70, 71, 73, 124
micro bcr (µ-bcr), 16

Index

minor bcr (m-bcr), 16
multiple myeloma, ix, 90, 91, 92, 93, 95, 105, 106, 107, 108, 121, 134
myelodysplasia, 48, 73, 116
myelodysplastic syndrome (MDS), vii, viii, ix, x, 8, 12, 14, 15, 23, 24, 32, 33, 34, 35, 36, 37, 42, 48, 51, 52, 59, 61, 62, 63, 69, 70, 73, 76, 79, 80, 81, 83, 84, 90, 91, 99, 101, 103, 111, 113, 114, 116, 120, 121, 123, 124, 126, 127, 128, 129, 133, 135
myelodysplastic syndromes, viii, 8, 14, 42, 51, 76, 79, 80, 81, 111, 126, 127, 128, 129, 133, 135
myelofibrosis, vii, 1, 4, 5, 6, 8, 13, 15, 38, 39, 42, 44, 46, 48
myeloid cells, x, 16, 114, 120
myeloproliferative disorders, 39, 42, 43

N

nausea, 64, 93, 95, 98, 100, 101
neoplasm, 22, 42, 47
neuroblastoma, 121, 134
neutropenia, 63, 64, 93, 99, 100
nicotinamide, 53, 76, 116, 118, 119
nuclear export, v, viii, 89, 90, 91, 92, 94, 102, 103, 104, 105, 106, 107, 108, 109, 110, 112
nuclear export inhibitors, 90, 110
nuclear membrane, 92
nuclear receptors, 28
nucleus, 3, 26, 27, 90, 92, 104, 117

O

olaparib, x, 72, 113, 114, 120, 121, 122, 123, 132, 133, 135, 136
oncogenes, viii, 2, 104, 116
oncoproteins, ix, 90, 91
opportunities, 77, 129, 136

P

p190, 16, 40
P210, 40
p230, 16, 40
pancreatic cancer, 105
PARP inhibitor, x, 71, 86, 87, 113, 114, 116, 118, 119, 120, 121, 122, 123, 125, 126, 130, 132, 133, 134, 135, 136, 137
PARP1 trapping, 114, 120, 125, 137
passenger mutations, 25, 29
pathogenesis, vii, 2, 26, 35, 37, 47, 79, 80, 96, 108, 115, 116, 126, 127, 128
pathway, x, 32, 48, 61, 66, 67, 68, 71, 75, 93, 113, 116, 118, 121, 131
PDGFRA (platelet derived growth factor receptor A), 22, 23, 42
PDGFRB (platelet derived growth factor receptor B), 22, 23
peripheral blood, vii, 1, 6, 8, 10, 12, 14, 15, 17, 18, 22, 23, 24
Philadelphia (Ph) chromosome, 17, 18, 19, 40
phosphorylation, 25, 27, 28, 46, 96, 124
poly(ADP-ribose) polymerase, v, vii, ix, 113, 114, 116, 117, 126, 130, 131, 136, 137
polycomb group proteins, 35
polycythemia, vii, 1, 4, 10, 11, 38, 39, 42, 44, 48
polycythemia vera (PV), vii, 1, 4, 9, 38, 39, 40, 42, 44, 48
primary myelofibrosis (PMF), vii, 1, 4, 5, 6, 7, 8, 9, 13, 14, 18, 23, 25, 26, 27, 28, 31, 32, 33, 34, 35, 36, 37, 38, 39, 42, 46, 48
progenitor cell, 31, 57, 80, 99, 127
prognosis, vii, viii, 2, 8, 16, 21, 22, 25, 41, 46, 47, 80, 82, 99, 115, 127, 134
proliferation, vii, 1, 3, 17, 28, 29, 33, 45, 61, 93, 108, 116, 117

proteins, ix, 3, 5, 6, 10, 14, 16, 25, 28, 30, 31, 33, 34, 36, 40, 43, 53, 89, 90, 91, 92, 93, 104, 106, 113, 117, 119
PV, vii, 1, 4, 7, 8, 9, 10, 11, 12, 14, 18, 23, 25, 26, 27, 32, 33, 34, 37, 79, 110

R

reactive oxygen, x, 57, 58, 114, 115, 135
receptor, viii, x, 26, 27, 28, 29, 44, 45, 46, 52, 89, 90, 93, 96, 100, 104, 114
recombination, x, 71, 86, 114, 115, 117, 118, 119, 120, 121, 122, 125, 126, 128, 133, 134
recommendations, iv, 41
recovery, 64, 65, 66, 68, 71, 86, 100, 101, 124, 130
remission, 12, 15, 60, 63, 64, 65, 66, 67, 70, 71, 82, 85, 97, 98, 99, 100, 101, 102, 111, 124
repair, x, 93, 106, 113, 114, 115, 116, 117, 118, 119, 120, 121, 122, 126, 127, 128, 130, 132, 133, 134, 135
resistance, ix, 20, 21, 41, 66, 70, 90, 91, 96, 101, 105, 108, 116, 128
response, viii, x, 6, 11, 12, 14, 15, 18, 19, 20, 21, 52, 61, 63, 64, 65, 66, 68, 69, 70, 85, 86, 94, 95, 96, 97, 98, 99, 100, 102, 109, 113, 114, 115, 116, 124, 127, 129, 132
ribose, vii, ix, 113, 114, 116, 117, 118, 126, 130, 131, 132, 133, 135, 136, 137
RUNX1, viii, x, 4, 24, 25, 33, 36, 49, 52, 65, 113, 121, 126

S

safety, 63, 66, 69, 70, 95, 96, 98, 101, 102

selinexor, vii, ix, 90, 91, 93, 94, 95, 96, 97, 98, 99, 100, 101, 102, 103, 106, 107, 108, 109, 110, 111
SETBP1, 4, 24, 43
SF3B1, 8, 24, 25, 35, 36, 43, 48
signaling pathway, 17, 21, 27, 29, 59, 62
somatic mutations, viii, 2, 25, 26, 46, 55, 73
SRSF2, 8, 24, 25, 35, 37, 48, 65, 73
stem cell differentiation, 30
stem cells, x, 3, 9, 61, 110, 113, 128
stratification, 38, 39, 40, 42, 74
survival, ix, 5, 22, 29, 30, 32, 39, 43, 58, 60, 61, 63, 65, 66, 68, 70, 71, 73, 90, 91, 95, 96, 98, 99, 101, 108, 123, 127
symptoms, 4, 6, 8, 9, 12, 13, 15, 17, 18, 22
syndrome, vii, ix, x, 7, 22, 40, 41, 48, 52, 64, 66, 67, 71, 83, 90, 91, 114, 127, 128, 129
synthesis, 58, 117, 120, 125, 137
synthetic lethality, 114, 117, 118, 122, 125, 126, 128, 134, 136

T

T618I, 29, 45
testing, 7, 10, 13, 23, 74, 136
TET2, 4, 7, 8, 12, 15, 23, 24, 25, 30, 31, 32, 33, 37, 46, 47, 57, 59, 65, 78, 79, 80, 122
therapeutic targets, 74
therapy, ix, 40, 42, 47, 60, 61, 63, 64, 65, 67, 68, 69, 71, 72, 73, 85, 90, 91, 96, 97, 98, 99, 101, 104, 105, 112, 116, 125, 128, 129, 134, 135
thrombocyte, 8, 17
thrombocytopenia, 6, 20, 93, 94, 95, 96, 98, 99, 101, 108
thrombocytosis, 14, 24, 43
thrombopoietin (TPO), 3, 26, 27, 28, 44, 108

transcription, viii, x, 18, 25, 30, 31, 36, 52, 92, 93, 113, 121, 131, 133, 134
transformation, 12, 15, 41, 46, 47, 60, 97
transport, viii, 54, 58, 89, 91, 104, 111
treatment, vii, viii, ix, x, 2, 3, 5, 7, 8, 11, 14, 17, 18, 20, 21, 23, 25, 32, 34, 39, 41, 42, 52, 61, 63, 64, 65, 66, 67, 68, 70, 71, 73, 74, 78, 83, 84, 90, 93, 95, 96, 98, 101, 105, 106, 107, 108, 110, 113, 124, 125, 136
trial, 63, 64, 67, 70, 72, 91, 94, 95, 98, 99, 100, 102, 103, 107, 108, 109, 111, 124, 125
triple negative, 8, 24
tumor, viii, ix, x, 2, 31, 34, 57, 58, 71, 72, 79, 84, 89, 91, 92, 93, 96, 100, 102, 112, 114, 122, 125, 136
tyrosine, viii, 9, 17, 20, 26, 27, 44, 52, 66, 100, 121, 134

U

U2AF1, 8, 25, 33, 35
ulcerative colitis, 22
unclassifiable MPNs (MPN-U), vii, 1, 4, 23, 24

V

V617F, 4, 7, 10, 11, 12, 15, 24, 25, 26, 43
vomiting, 93, 98, 100, 101

W

W515, 27, 44
weakness, 5, 6, 9, 13, 17
weight loss, 9, 17, 24, 91